# Workbook on Renal Replacement Therapy in ICU

ISCCM
PUNE BRANCH

# Workbook on Renal Replacement Therapy in ICU

***Editors***

**Valentine Lobo** MD DNB (Nephrology)
Consultant Nephrologist
King Edward Memorial Hospital
Pune, Maharashtra, India

**Sunitha Binu Varghese** DNB (Medicine) IDCCM EDIC FICCM
Head, Department of Critical Care
Niramaya Hospital
Pune, Maharashtra, India

**Jignesh N Shah** MD DNB (Anesthesiology) IDCCM IFCCM EDIC
Associate Professor
Department of Critical Care
Bharati Vidyapeeth Deemed University
Medical College and Bharati Hospital
Pune, Maharashtra, India

***Foreword***

**Shirish Prayag**

ISCCM
PUNE BRANCH

JAYPEE

JAYPEE BROTHERS MEDICAL PUBLISHERS
*The Health Sciences Publisher*
New Delhi | London

**Jaypee Brothers Medical Publishers (P) Ltd**

**Headquarters**
EMCA House
23/23-B, Ansari Road, Daryaganj
New Delhi 110 002, India
Landline: +91-11-23272143, +91-11-23272703
+91-11-23282021, +91-11-23245672
E-mail: jaypee@jaypeebrothers.com

**Corporate Office**
Jaypee Brothers Medical Publishers (P) Ltd.
4838/24, Ansari Road, Daryaganj
New Delhi 110 002, India
Phone: +91-11-43574357
Fax: +91-11-43574314
E-mail: jaypee@jaypeebrothers.com

**Overseas Office**
JP Medical Ltd.
83, Victoria Street, London
SW1H 0HW (UK)
Phone: +44-20 3170 8910
E-mail: info@jpmedpub.com

**EU GPSR** Authorised Representative
Logos Europe, 9 rue Nicolas Poussin
17000, La Rochelle, France
Phone: +33 (0) 6 67 93 73 78
E-mail: Contact@logoseurope.eu

Website: www.jaypeebrothers.com
Website: www.jaypeedigital.com



**Inquiries for bulk sales may be solicited at**: jaypee@jaypeebrothers.com

***Workbook on Renal Replacement Therapy in ICU***

*First Edition:* 2020, *Reprint:* ***2026***

ISBN: 978-93-89188-42-4

*Printed in India by Replika Press Pvt. Ltd.*

# CONTRIBUTORS

**Ashutosh Garg** MBBS MD
Principal Consultant Intensive Care
Max Superspeciality Hospital
Patparganj, New Delhi, India

**Jignesh N Shah**
MD DNB (Anesthesiology) IDCCM IFCCM EDIC
Associate Professor
Department of Critical Care
Bharati Vidyapeeth Deemed University Medical College and Bharati Hospital
Pune, Maharashtra, India

**Juliet Merlene**
MSc Nursing (Critical Care) BSC Nursing, PGDEM
Lead Clinical and Field trainer-Renal Acute
Baxter India Pvt Ltd
DLF Cyber City, DLF Phase-II
Gurugram, Haryana, India

**Jyothsna G** MBBS, MD (AB)
Consultant Nephrologist
Star Hospitals
Hyderabad, Telangana, India

**Kapil Zirpe**
MBBS MD (Chest) FICCM FCCM
Director
Neurotrauma Unit
Ruby Hall Clinic
Pune, Maharashtra, India

**Kayanoosh J Kadapatti**
MD DNB (Medicine) IDCCM EDIC
Consultant and Head
Department of Intensive Care
Jehangir Hospital
Pune, Maharashtra, India

**Pradeep D'Costa** DNB (Medicine)
ICU-in-charge
King Edward Memorial Hospital, Pune
Intensivist Physician
Sahyadri Hospital (Nagar Road Branch)
Pune, Maharashtra, India

**Rajasekara Chakravarthi M** MBBS MD DNB
Consultant Nephrologist
Star Hospitals
Hyderabad, Telangana, India

**Rajeev A Annigeri** MBBS MD DNB
Senior Nephrology Consultant
Apollo Hospitals
Chennai, Tamil Nadu, India

**Ranajit Chatterjee**
MBBS MRCPI (DUBLIN) EDICM DA (Gold Medal)
Chief Medical Officer (NFSG)
In-charge Accident and Emergency
In-charge Intensive Care
Swami Dayanand Hospital, New Delhi, India

**Sachin S Soni** MD DNB (Nephrology)
Consultant Interventional Nephrology
United Ciigma Hospital
Aurangabad, Maharashtra, India.

**Shriganesh R Barnela** MD DNB (Nephrology)
Consultant Interventional Nephrology
United Ciigma Hospital
Aurangabad, Maharashtra, India

**Siddhesh Dhaygude**
DNB (Medicine) DNB (Nephrology)
Consultant Nephrologist
King Edward Memorial Hospital, Pune
Niramaya Hospital, Chinchwad
Sterling Hospital
Nigdi, Maharashtra, India

**Snehal Gaikwad** MBBS MD Medicine, DNB Nephrology
Consultant Nephrologist
King Edward Memorial Hospital
Pune, Maharashtra, India

**Sonali S Saboo** DMRD DNB (Radiodiagnosis)
Consultant Radiologist
United Ciigma Hospital
Aurangabad, Maharashtra, India

**Sunil Karanth** MD (Int Medicine), FNB (Critical Care Medicine) EDIC FCICM (Aus/NZ)
Chairman
Critical Care Services
Manipal Health Enterprises (P) Ltd
Adjunct Professor, Critical Care Medicine
Manipal University, Manipal Hospital
Bengaluru, Karnataka, India

**Sunitha Binu Varghese** DNB (Medicine) IDCCM EDIC
Head, Department of Critical Care
Niramaya Hospital
Pune, Maharashtra, India

**Suresh H Saboo** DMRD MD (Radiodiagnosis)
Professor of Radiology
JIIU's Indian Institute of
Medical Sciences and Research
Aurangabad, Maharashtra, India

**Sushma Gurav** MBBS DA DNB (Anesthesiology)
Postgraduation in Medicolegal Concepts
Consultant, Neurotrauma Unit
Ruby Hall Clinic
Pune, Maharashtra, India

**Tarun K Jeloka** MD DM FICN FASN FRCP
Associate Director
Aditya Birla Memorial Hospital
Pune, Maharashtra, India

**Unmesh V Takalkar** MS (General Surgery)
Consultant Laparoscopy and GI Surgery
United Ciigma Hospital
Aurangabad, Maharashtra, India

**Valentine Lobo** MD DNB (Nephrology)
Consultant Nephrologist
King Edward Memorial Hospital
Pune, Maharashtra, India

**Venkatesh Dhat** MBBS DA DNB IDCCM ICU
Consultant
Aditya Birla Memorial Hospital
Pune, Maharashtra, India

**Vijay Varma P** MBBS MD DM
Consultant Nephrologist, Star Hospitals,
Hyderabad, Telangana, India

**Vipul Chakurkar** MD DNB (Nephrology)
Jr Consultant Nephrologist
King Edward Memorial Hospital
Pune, Maharashtra, India

**Vishwanath C Patil**
MD (Anesthesiology) IDCCM, IFCCM EDIC
Assistant Professor, Critical Care Medicine
Bharati Vidyapeeth Deemed University
Medical College and Bharati Hospital
Pune, Maharashtra, India

# FOREWORD

It is with a great degree of pleasure and pride that I am writing this Foreword.

Although isolated foci of excellence in critical care existed in India in individual centers 25 years ago, there was no organized professional activity. Training in this evolving field was nonexistent. It was then in 1992, that an organized platform for discussions in small group was started in Pune, Maharashtra, India under the banner of Critical Care Society. In 1993, the National Indian Society of Critical Care Medicine (ISCCM) was born and this local activity in Pune merged with ISCCM as its first city branch.

Over the last almost 25 years of activity, Pune Branch of ISCCM has remained in the forefront of academic activities of ISCCM and the critical care world in India. There have been innumerable activities, and all this has led to Pune being awarded the Best Branch award for many consecutive years.

We have always believed in giving something different, unique and enriching to the world of critical care in India. The workbooks for various workshops are therefore a part of this continuing process of dynamic output from this branch.

The field of Renal Replacement Therapy (RRT) represents the robust growth as well as the dilemmas of the field of critical care medicine. Initially, we started by doing peritoneal dialysis. As the hemodialysis machines became more easily available, the field of RRT has boomed. Continuous renal replacement therapy (CRRT) machines evolved soon and gradually in ICUs, the decisions regarding the RRT became easier to critical care physicians and nephrologists. This science has erupted and this workshop is an indicator of how much we need to know about these techniques.

All this and much more is discussed in this important workbook. The contributions have come from many national specialists of repute in the field of critical care medicine and nephrology. The topics that are discussed are extremely practical, relevant, and important for day-to-day practice to all those who spend majority of their time with clinical work.

This book fulfills an important lacuna in the field of critical care medicine in India. That void was due to the need of a practical workbook in the field of RRT for critically ill patients. I am sure that practising intensivists will find it a worthwhile addition.

I look forward to ISCCM Pune branch continuing to make many such praiseworthy contributions.

**Shirish Prayag**
MD FCCM
Director, Critical Care
Prayag Hospital
Pune, Maharashtra, India

# PREFACE

In 1946, Wilhem Kolff first used the rotating drum dialyzer to save the life of a patient with acute kidney injury (AKI) and the mortality of this condition decreased by 50%. The subsequent seven decades have seen profound advances in the fields of Nephrology and Critical Care, yet the mortality of patients with AKI remains around 50%.

One reason for this unchanged mortality is the fact that AKI is more often a part of multiorgan failure rather than occurring in isolation. With improvements in infection control, surgery and obstetrics, and increased use of interventional radiology procedures, patients admitted to the ICU are older, have more comorbidities, survive the initial disease more often, and are subjected to more nephrotoxic treatments as a part of life saving therapy. Unsurprisingly the incidence of AKI in critically ill patients has increased and has been shown unequivocally to increase mortality. Around 6% of such patients require renal replacement therapy and have an expected mortality of around 60–75%, a distressingly high rate.

While elegant studies have advanced our knowledge and the care of patients with septic shock and acute respiratory distress syndrome (ARDS), several questions remain unanswered about providing renal replacement therapy in an ICU, including the optimum modality, dose and timing of RRT, though some light now appears visible at the end of the tunnel. An equal cause of concern is that cost and lack of infrastructure have hampered the growth of Critical Care Nephrology in India, at a rate commensurate with advances in other fields of critical care and hindered the efforts of those intensivists and nephrologists who would like to see it advance faster. A boost has been given to our efforts by the demonstration in observational studies that previously used but forgotten therapies like peritoneal dialysis have a life-saving role and a revival of interest may be seen in these modalities.

This workbook and the workshop run by the Pune Indian Society of Critical Care Medicine (ISCCM) branch are an attempt to fill the existing gaps and provide an adequate knowledge for intensivists and nephrologists to provide the most appropriate renal replacement therapy in their individual ICUs. A group of nephrologists and intensivists many of whom have started as pioneers and emerged as experts in the field have combined to put together the subsequent chapters in this book. It has been a pleasure to collate their efforts and we sincerely hope that our readers would find it useful.

We as editors are grateful to all contributors and those who provided us feedback in the run up to this effort. This is not an attempt to write another textbook, several of which exist on the subject. Rather we hope to provide practical points which would assist the intensivist caring for patients with AKI a roadmap to RRT and to provide the nephrologist whose training has not exposed him to the vulnerable patient in the ICU an understanding of the special needs of such a patient. We firmly believe that the "two" need to work closely in collaboration to provide the best care and outcomes for their patients and make "0by25" initiative a reality.

Finally we dedicate this effort to our teachers, from whom we have learned a lot, our students and colleagues from whom we learned more, and our patients without whom we would not have "gone to sea at all". A special mention must also be made of the efforts of our dialysis and intensive care nurses and technicians whom John Kellum rightly called the unsung heroes of critical care renal replacement therapy.

**Valentine Lobo**
**Sunitha Binu Varghese**
**Jignesh N Shah**

# ACKNOWLEDGMENTS

On behalf of Indian Society of Critical Care Medicine Pune Branch, I acknowledge our editors who have worked tirelessly to complete this outstanding Workbook on Renal Replacement Therapy. I also sincerely appreciate each and every author for their valuable contribution and timely completion of the chapters.

Everyone's efforts, dedication, and experience are evident in the quality of the book.

I am confident that this book will meet its desired goal of providing practical knowledge on Renal Replacement Therapy that will improve patient outcome. I look forward to see more such activities in future which will lead to improvement in patient care.

I am grateful to the office bearers and members of the Pune branch of the Indian Society of Critical Care Medicine for the continuous support received throughout our efforts, to our publishers especially Jaypee Brothers Medical Publishers Pvt. Ltd., New Delhi, India and to the companies who provide us the cutting edge technology in this field.

**Jyoti Shendge**

Chairman, ISCCM Pune Branch

# CONTENTS

# PLATE 1

## CHAPTER 1

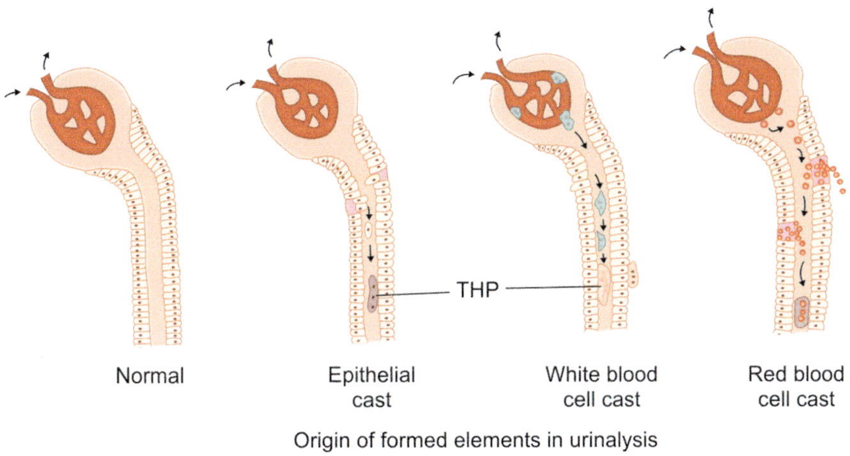


**Fig. 2:** Origin of formed elements in urinalysis.
(THP: Tamm–Horsfall protein)

## CHAPTER 3

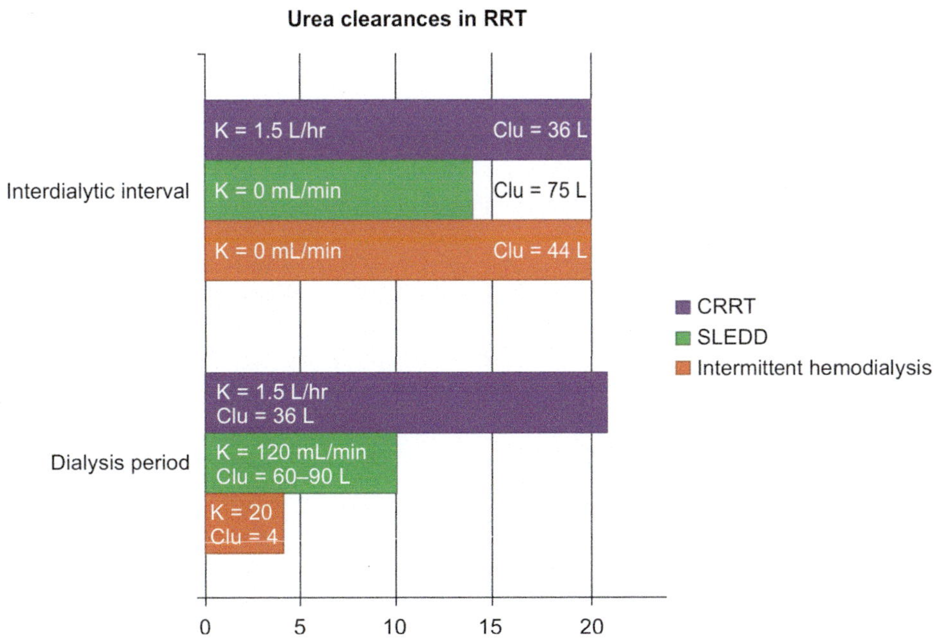


**Fig. 4:** Effects of dialytic and interdialytic time on clearance.
(CRRT: continuous renal replacement therapy; SLEDD: slow low-efficiency extended daily dialysis; Clu: urea clearance))

## CHAPTER 4

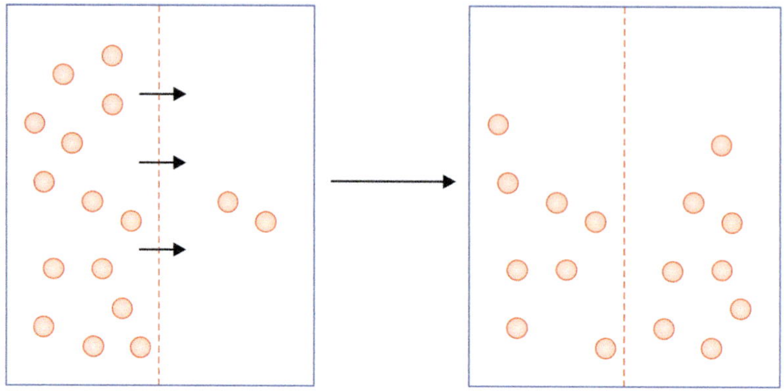

Movement of solutes form high to low concentration across a semipermeable membrane

**Fig. 1:** Diffusion.

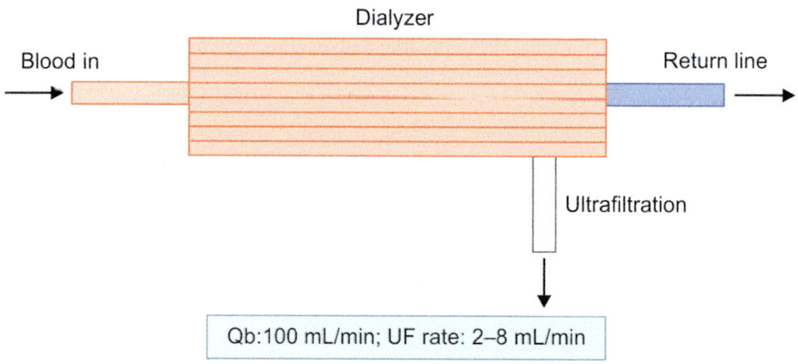


**Fig. 2:** Slow continuous ultrafiltration.

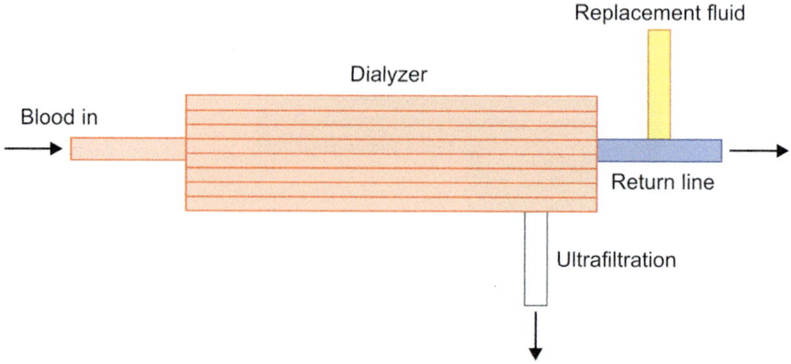


**Fig. 3:** Continuous venovenous hemofiltration.
(UF: ultrafiltration)

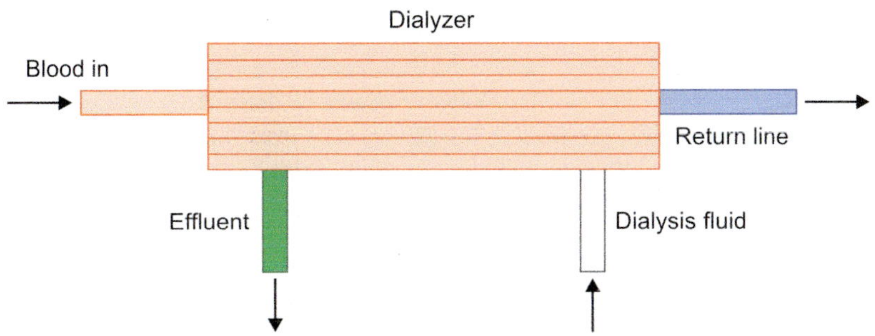


**Fig. 4:** Continuous venovenous hemodialysis.

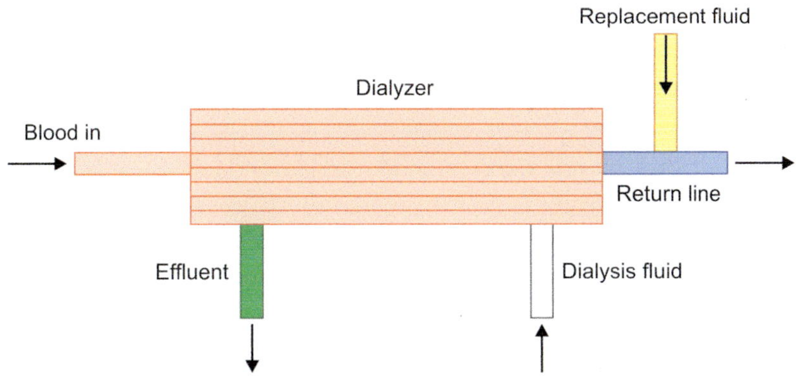


**Fig. 5:** Continuous venovenous hemodiafiltration.

## CHAPTER 6

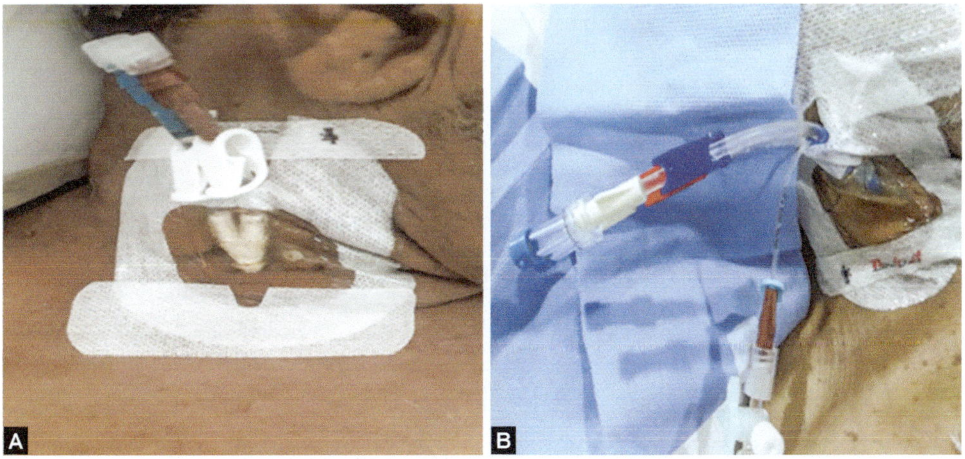


**Figs. 1A and B:** Temporary/nontunneled catheter—double-lumen and triple-lumen catheters.

## CHAPTER 8

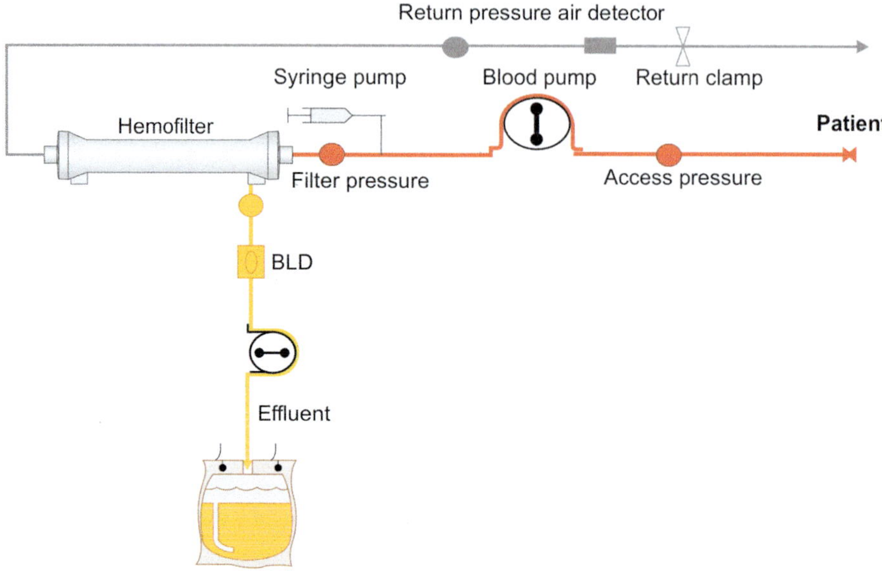


**Fig. 1:** Slow continuous ultrafiltration.

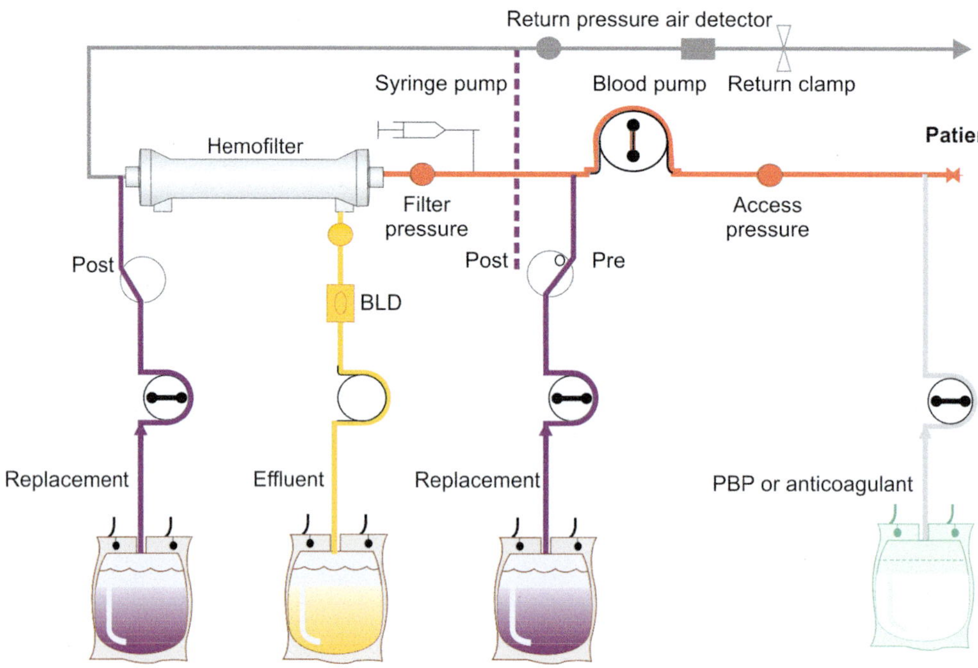


**Fig. 2:** Continuous venovenous hemofiltration.

# PLATE 5

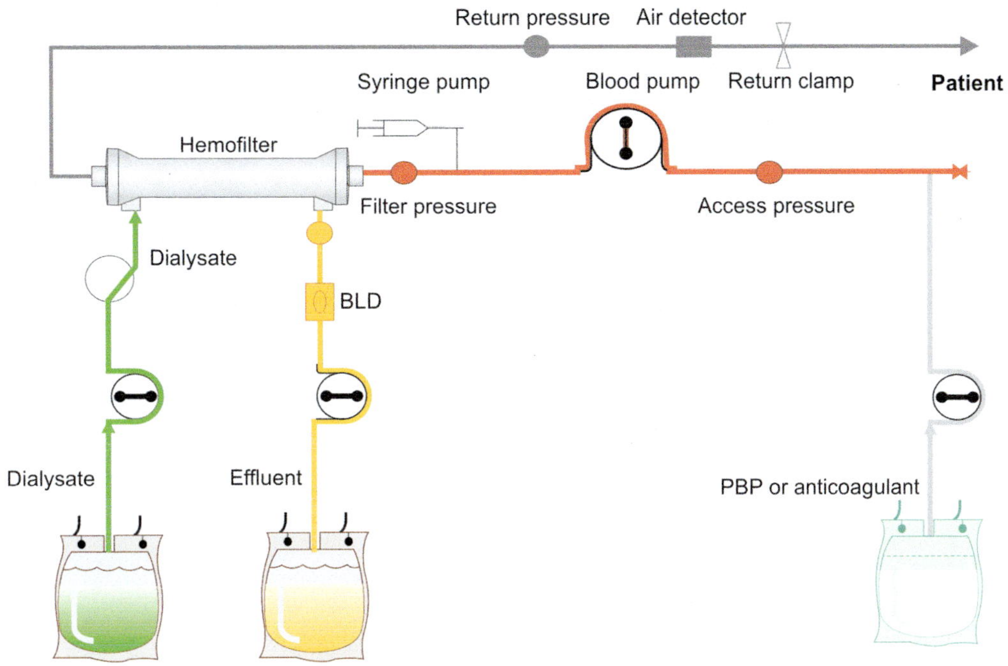


**Fig. 3:** Continuous venovenous hemodialysis.

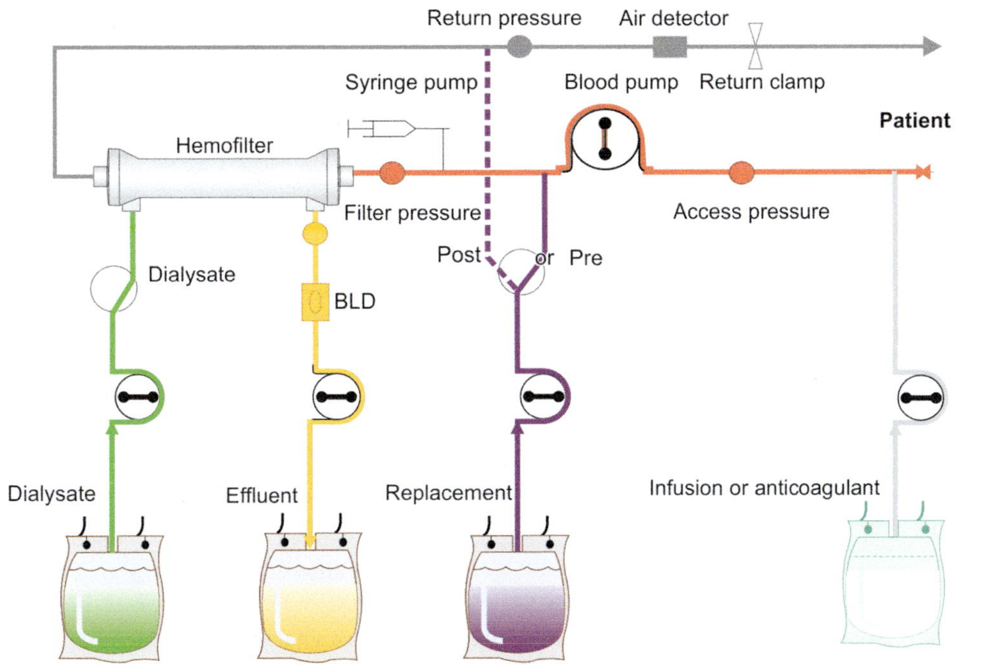


**Fig. 4:** Continuous venovenous hemodiafiltration.

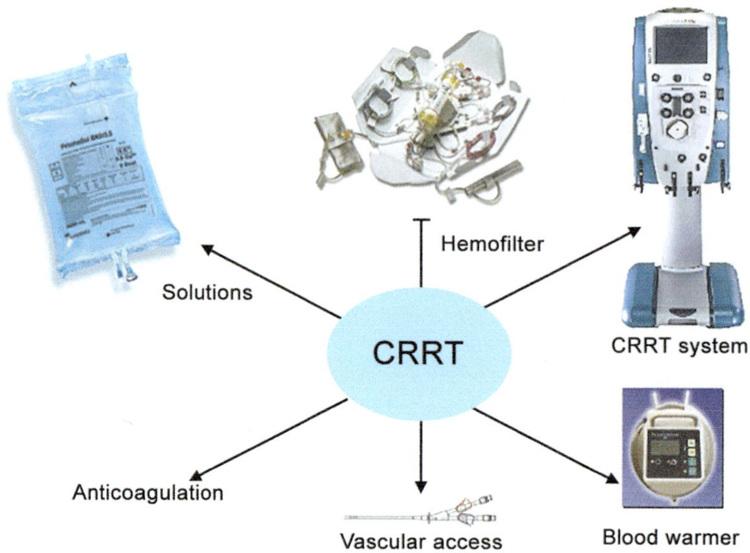


**Fig. 5:** Components of CRRT.

## CHAPTER 16

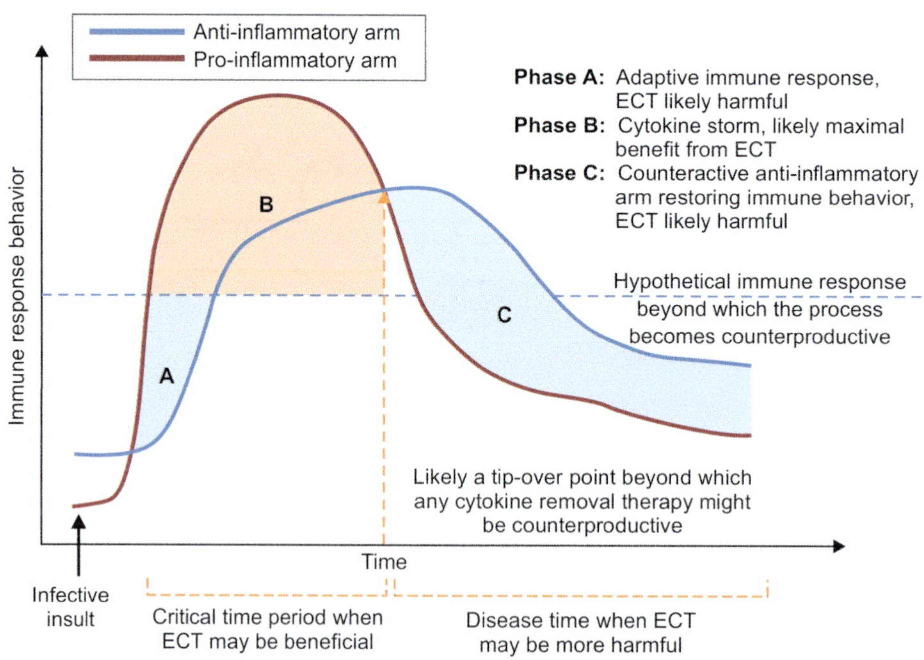


**Fig. 1:** Theoretical considerations of the likely impact of ECT in a single-hit model of sepsis, and its correlation to the stage and severity of disease.

(ECT: extracorporeal therapy)

CHAPTER 1

# Acute Kidney Injury: Definition, Classification, Diagnostic Strategies, and Prevention

*Kayanoosh J Kadapatti*

## INTRODUCTION

Till recently there was no standard definition for acute renal failure (ARF). In 1993, the late Roger Bone penned the following words:

*"Too often, the way we describe a disorder influences, and often limits, the way we think about that disorder".*

## DEFINITION

The term "acute kidney injury" is intended to emphasize the reversible nature of most renal insults. ARF is a terminology now reserved for kidney injury that necessitates renal replacement therapy (RRT) (i.e. any method of conventional or intermittent dialysis).

Clinically, acute kidney injury (AKI) is characterized by a rapid reduction in kidney function resulting in failure to maintain:

- Fluid and electrolyte
- Acid–base homeostasis
- Inability to excrete nitrogenous wastes.

It is not an innocent bystander reflecting coexistent pathologies but is an independent predictor of mortality. AKI is common affecting 5–10% of hospitalized patients and up to 60% of patients admitted to the intensive care units (ICUs).

Medical understanding of AKI has been augmented by the RIFLE criteria coined by the Acute Dialysis Quality Initiative (ADQI) group in 2007. The acronym "RIFLE" classifies renal dysfunction according to the degree of impairment present: risk (R), injury (I), and failure (F), sustained loss (L) and end-stage kidney disease (E). The staging is based on the serum creatinine and the urine output criteria. If the urine output and the creatinine do not correspond to the same stage then the higher stage should be considered.

The RIFLE criteria incorporated three categories of injury and two outcomes that varied in severity. Subsequent definitions by Acute Kidney Injury Network (AKIN) and Kidney Disease Improving Global Outcomes (KDIGO) by 2012 eliminated the outcomes, i.e. loss and end-stage kidney disease (ESKD). The AKIN definition used smaller changes in serum creatinine to stage the degree of injury while the KDIGO added more definitive timelines to their criteria (Table 1).

The AKIN definition incorporated smaller changes in serum creatinine (SCr) concentration, and the KDIGO definition added more definitive time frames to the definition. A key concept for the SCr-based definitions of AKI is the identification of baseline SCr concentration. Although the initial RIFLE criteria recommended the use of an Scr concentration that would equate to estimated glomerular filtration rate (eGFR) of 75 mL/min/1.73 m$^2$ by the Modification of Diet in Renal Disease (MDRD) study equation (MDRD-75) if no baseline was available, this definition does not account for chronic kidney disease if present. It is essential to look for a prior baseline/reference SCr concentration, ideally from the 365 days before hospital admission from a clinical context in which there was no concern for AKI (e.g. a stable clinic visit) (Table 2).

**Table 1:** Comparison of classification systems for AKI.

| *Stage of AKI* | *Urine output* | *KDIGO* | *AKIN* | *RIFLE* |
|---|---|---|---|---|
| 1 | < 0.5 mL/kg/hr for 6–12 hours | Rise of serum creatinine 1.5–1.9 × baseline over 7 days or ≥0.3 mg/dL absolute increase over 48 hours | Rise of serum creatinine 1.5–2 × baseline or ≥0.3 mg/dL absolute increase over 48 hours | *Risk*: Rise of s creatinine ≥1.5 × increase within 7 days, sustained for ≥24 hours |
| 2 | <0.5 mL/kg/hr for >12 hours | Serum creatinine 2–2.9 × baseline | Serum creatinine 2–3 x baseline | *Injury*: Serum creatinine ≥2 × increase |
| 3 | <0.3 mL/kg/hr for ≥24 hours or anuria for ≥12 hours | Serum creatinine to ≥3 × baseline or serum creatinine increase to 4.0 mg/dL or initiation of RRT | Serum creatinine to >3 × baseline or serum creatinine increase to ≥4.0 mg/dL (with increase of 0.5 mg/dL) or initiation of RRT | *Failure*: Serum creatinine to ≥3 × increase or serum creatinine increase to ≥4.0 mg/dL (with increase of 0.5mg/dL) or initiation of RRT |
| | | | | *Loss*: Complete loss of kidney function for >4 weeks |
| | | | | *ESKD*: ESKD for >3 months |

(AKI: acute kidney injury; AKIN: Acute Kidney Injury Network; ESKD: end-stage kidney disease; KDIGO: Kidney Disease Improving Global Outcomes; RRT: renal replacement therapy)

**Table 2:** Application of the RIFLE to AKI in 24 studies including 71,000 patients.

| *Comparison of AKI levels* | *Mortality* | *RR (95% CI)* | *P-value* |
|---|---|---|---|
| Non-AKI | 6.9% | 1 | – |
| Risk vs non-AKI | 18.9% | 2.4 (1.94–2.97) | <0.00001 |
| Injury vs non-AKI | 36.1% | 4.2 (3.14–5.48) | <0.0001 |
| Failure vs non-AKI | 46.5% | 6.37 (5.14–7.9) | <0.0001 |
| Injury vs risk | – | 1.51 (1.23–1.86) | <0.0001 |
| Failure vs risk | – | 2.24 (1.79–2.8) | <0.0001 |
| Failure vs injury | – | 1.45 (1.25–1.69) | <0.0001 |

Overall 30-day mortality in patients requiring RRT was 56.1% in one study and 76% in another.
(AKI: acute kidney injury; CI: confidence interval; RR: relative risk)

The KDIGO-AKI definition validation was done by Rodrigues et al. 2013. It was a prospective study of 1,050 people in first 7 days after hospitalization with acute myocardial infarction (AMI). AKI defined by RIFLE in 14.8% and KDIGO 36.6% patients were associated with increased 30-day and 1-year death rate. People diagnosed as not having AKI by RIFLE, but AKI by KDIGO had increased risk of death or CKD.

## MODIFICATION OF KDIGO—ADQI 16 FOR DEVELOPING COUNTRIES

Persistent AKI is characterized by the continuance of AKI by creatinine or urine output criteria (defined by KDIGO criteria) beyond 48 hours from onset. Acute kidney disease (AKD) is defined as a condition wherein AKI Stage I or greater criteria is present 7 days (or more) after an exposure. AKD that persists beyond 90 days is then considered CKD.

A Prospective Indian Study of 316 patients in 1 year evaluating the clinical profile and correlation of patients with AKI according to the KDIGO definition with respect to incidence outcome and different causes of AKI concluded that AKI is an independent risk factor for mortality in ICU. It showed that AKI is present in 37.7% of ICU patients and 9.1% patients developed AKI in ICU. The KDIGO staging could not predict outcomes because of multisystem failure.

## KDIGO DEFINITION APPLICABILITY

If the urine output and the SCr do not correspond to the same stage then the higher stage should be considered.

Patients who develop AKI by KDIGO urine output criteria regardless of whether serum creatinine criteria present are at risk of developing fluid overload given the typical high obligate intake of critically ill patients.

Since creatinine lags acute changes in kidney function, the current AKI stage may not reflect current kidney function. There could be reductions in creatinine production due to acute illness, sarcopenia, and creatinine dilution during volume overload complicating evaluation of kidney function. AKI does not obey steady state kinetics for calculation of GFR.

## ACUTE KIDNEY INJURY—INCIDENCE AND MORTALITY

About 25–30% of admissions to ICU are complicated by AKI, mostly as part of multiple organ dysfunction syndrome (MODS). Like acute respiratory distress syndrome it represents a syndrome rather than a single disease entity. Mortality of ARF in the ICU is 72% and non ICU-ARF is 32%. Mortality of ARF associated with acute respiratory failure is approximately 90%. Thus one must aim to prevent AKI from progressing to ARF (Fig. 1).

*A special mention with regard to rhabdomyolysis in this context*: It is a cause of 5–10% of ICU-ARF in a multicenter series, mostly because of trauma, muscle injury, narcotic overdose, and vascular blockade. Comorbid conditions are often present and one-third of the patients may have underlying renal disease. Early detection and aggressive renal support may improve survival by 30%

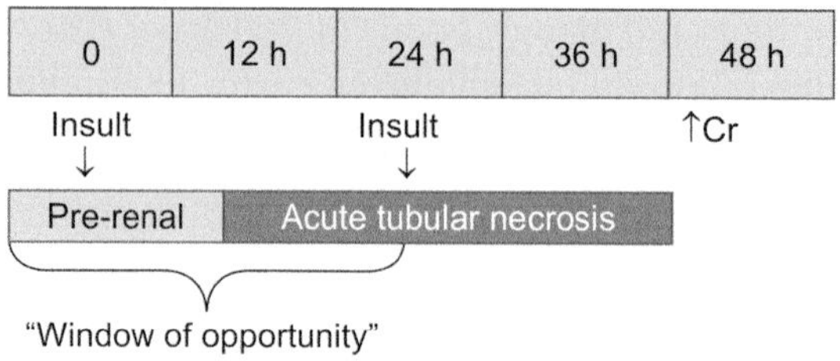


**Fig. 1:** Progression from pre-renal to acute tubular necrosis.

## DIAGNOSTIC STRATEGIES IN AKI (FLOWCHART 1)

- Careful history is essential
- Physical examination
- *Blood investigations*:
  - Serum creatinine level—compare
  - Complete blood count
  - Newer biomarkers
- Urinalysis and urine electrolytes
- Imaging studies
- Renal biopsy.

### Role of Biomarkers in Diagnosis of AKI

Serum creatinine levels have poor sensitivity and specificity in AKI, slowing recognition and its therapeutic management. Biomarkers like neutrophil gelatinase-associated lipocalin, kidney injury molecule-1, interleukin-18, and liver-type fatty acid-binding protein (L-FABP) show promise for representing the "troponin-like" molecule of AKI. Biomarkers that reflect kidney stress like tissue injury metalloproteinase 2 (TIMP 2) and insulin-like growth factor binding protein 7 (IGFBP 7) have been recently approved by the US Food and Drug Administration for identifying patients at high risk for developing KDIGO stage 2 and 3 AKI during the next 12–24 hours. These are marketed as NephroCheck test (Astute Medical). Thus if renal injury can be diagnosed sooner in its etiologic process, therapeutic interventions can be instituted more promptly, thereby improving secondary disease prevention.

#### *Pitfalls of Biomarkers*

- Biomarkers are released at a specific time point—the rise in levels is temporary
- Cut-off levels show disparity
- Comparison with urine output and creatinine
- Real-time measurements of glomerular filtration have not been used in assessment.

**Flowchart 1:** Diagnostic strategies in acute kidney injury (AKI).

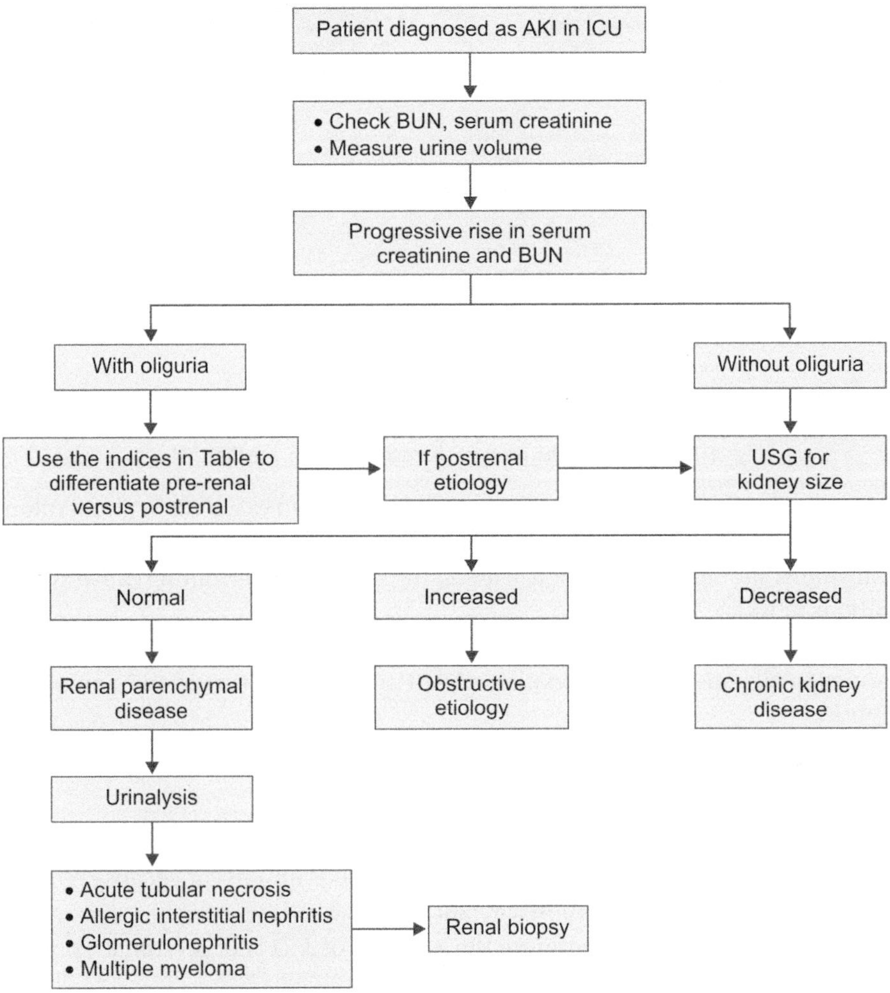


(BUN: blood urea nitrogen; ICU: intensive care unit; USG: ultrasonography)

## Urinalysis and Urine Electrolytes

It is not quite fair to say that creatinine is the only biomarker of AKI. Urinalysis is a very helpful test for identifying evidence of kidney damage. Ordinarily there are very few formed elements in the urine. However, after AKI, renal epithelial cells can be shed into the tubular lumen and detected in the urine. Furthermore, these can form renal epithelial cell casts when they gel with Tamm–Horsfall protein that is present in everyone's urine. Other elements in the urinary tract can also form casts, including white blood cells that might indicate infection and red blood cells, which typically indicate glomerular inflammation (Fig. 2).

If urine dipstick is positive for blood or white cells urine should be sent for urgent microscopy for casts as well as for culture.

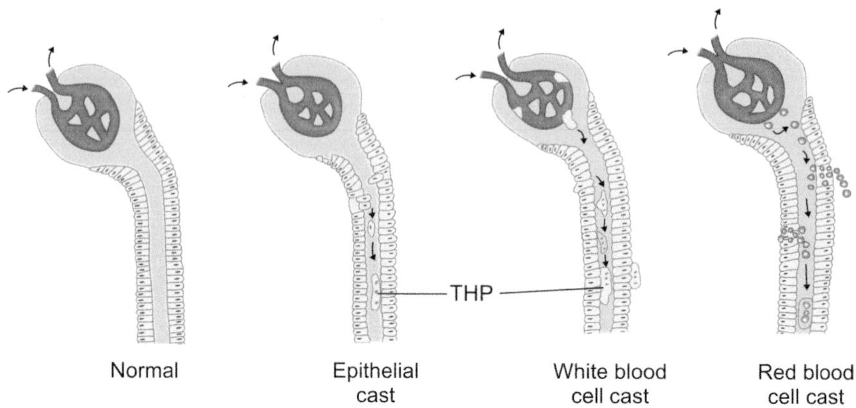


**Fig. 2:** Origin of formed elements in urinalysis.
(THP: Tamm–Horsfall protein) *(For color version, see Plate 1)*

*Renal biopsy* should be reserved for patients with suspected vasculitis or glomerulonephritis (GN), especially if a trial of steroids are considered.

Investigations should also be aimed at assessing severity, determining cause and detecting complications of AKI.

*Renal ultrasound and/or a plain computed tomography of kidneys, ureters and bladder* should be performed in all patients with unexplained ARF to exclude obstruction or emphysematous pyelonephritis.

## ANATOMICAL CLASSIFICATION OF AKI (FIG. 3)

Once a diagnosis of AKI has been established, it is important to stratify the patient's condition by etiology (i.e. pre renal, renal, or post-renal). Stratification is important because recommended therapeutic models are tailored to these categories (Fig. 3).

General guidelines for differentiating the etiology of AKI (i.e. pre-renal vs. renal) using laboratory studies can be used (Table 3).

It is important to identify and treat the treatable factors. This involves hemodynamic resuscitation, relief of obstruction, including urinary retention, antibiotics and aggressive source control for sepsis, stopping nephrotoxic drugs where possible, decompression of abdominal compartment syndrome, and treatment of rhabdomyolysis (Table 4).

## PREVENTION OF AKI

### Appropriate Adequate Aggressive Volume Resuscitation

As per the Surviving Sepsis Campaign guidelines keep central venous pressure (CVP) at 8–12 mm Hg, mean arterial pressure (MAP) around 65 mm Hg, $SVO_2$ of >70%, and maintain a urine output of 0.5–1.0 mL/kg/hr. To avoid organ edema do not over-resuscitate. Colloids or crystalloids may be equally effective but recommended is crystalloid 30 mL/kg over first 3

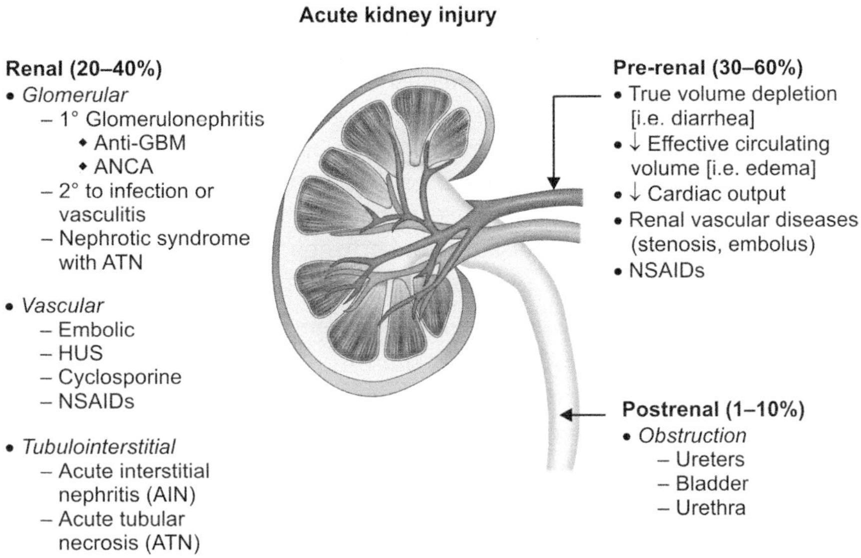


**Fig. 3:** Anatomical classification of acute kidney injury.
(HUS: hemolytic-uremic syndrome; NSAIDs: nonsteroidal anti-inflammatory drugs)

**Table 3:** Helpful indices to differentiate pre-renal from renal causes.

| *Indices* | *Pre-renal* | *Renal* |
|---|---|---|
| Blood urea nitrogen to creatinine ratio | >20 | <20 |
| Fraction of filtered sodium % | <1 | >2 |
| Fractional excretion of urea | <35 | >35 |
| Urine osmolality mOsm/L | >500 | <400 |
| Urine sediment cast type | Bland, hyaline | Granular |
| Urine sodium mEq/L | <20 | >40 |

**Table 4:** Treatable factors to prevent progression of AKI.

| *Condition* | *Treatment strategy* |
|---|---|
| Hypovolemia and shock | Volume repletion with serial fluid challenges monitoring IVC collapsibility index or trend of CVP |
| | Restore blood pressure (MAP) and cardiac output with vasopressors/inotropes if other evidence of tissue hypoperfusion—may need MAP >80 mm Hg if previously hypertensive |
| Infection | Source control and antibiotics |
| Nephrotoxic drugs | Identify and discontinue where possible |
| Abdominal compartment syndrome | Decompress |
| Rhabdomyolysis | Alkalinize, mannitol |
| Obstruction | Catheterize, DJ stenting |

(AKI: acute kidney injury; CVP: central venous pressure; IVC: inferior vena cava; MAP: mean arterial pressure)

hours. High and medium molecular weight starches are to be avoided as they can cause osmotic nephropathy.

Vasoactive agents may be used simultaneously with volume resuscitation to restore the MAP to >65 mm Hg. Noradrenaline is the first choice to correct hypotension. Dobutamine is an inotropic agent that stimulates beta receptors and results in increased cardiac output. In theory, it can enhance tissue oxygen delivery in patients with septic shock who have received adequate fluid resuscitation and vasopressor support. In early goal-directed therapy (EGDT), dobutamine is recommended if there is evidence of tissue hypoperfusion [central venous oxygen saturation ($ScvO_2$) < 70 mm Hg] after CVP, MAP, and hematocrit goals have been met.

*Low-dose dopamine should not be used for renal protection*

Dopamine has an inconsistent diuretic effect but this may cause dehydration. It does not increase creatinine clearance or prevent ARF but may cause serious toxicity problems like tachyarrhythmias, exacerbating renal, and mesenteric ischemia, impairing immune function. It should thus fundamentally not be used as an inotrope or in renal dose. Two meta-analyses of 22 trials involving 970 patients showed no benefit.

*Furosemide* seems to reduce juxtamedullary oxygen consumption and adds the advantage of easier maintenance of fluid and electrolyte balance by converting oliguric to nonoliguric renal failure. But it does not improve creatinine clearance or affect survival either way. It may be used but *ONLY* after adequate volume resuscitation. It does not prevent the development of acute tubular necrosis (ATN) and there is no reduction in mortality or need for dialysis. Furosemide is *NOT* a resuscitation fluid.

## Nonpharmacologic Strategies for Prevention

- *Minimize nephrotoxin exposure*:
  - Candidate agents—aminoglycosides, amphotericin B, nonsteroidal anti-inflammatory drugs (NSAIDs), and radiocontrast media
  - Once daily gentamicin vs thrice daily dosing has equal efficacy but lower toxicity—5% vs 24%.
- *Avoid nephrotoxic combinations*: Use of NSAIDs and aminoglycoside in postoperative diabetic patients is a common clinical scenario which predisposes a patient to drug-induced AKI (Box 1).
- *Adjust doses proportional to the creatinine clearance/eGFR*: GFR is considered the gold standard for estimating acute or chronic renal function. GFR is almost never directly measured in the clinical setting and is almost always calculated. Current eGFR equations like Cockcroft and Gault [140-(Age × weight)/serum creatinine × 72], MDRD study, and CKD Epidemiology Collaboration (CKD-EPI),

**Box 1: Nephrotoxic agents.**

*Nephrotoxic agents associated with acute tubular necrosis*

- Acyclovir
- Aminoglycosides (tobramycin and gentamycin)
- Amphotericin B
- Benzoylmethyl ecognine (cocaine)
- Cisplatin
- Cyclosporine
- Foscarnet sodium
- Highly active antiretroviral therapy
- Intravenous immunoglobulin therapy
- Medical contrast media, e.g. hyperosmolar radiocontrast media
- Nonsteroidal anti-inflammatory drugs (Ibuprofen, naproxen, ketorolac, and celecoxib)
- Penicillins
- Tacrolimus
- Zoledronic acid
- Angiotensin-converting enzyme inhibitor/Angiotensin-receptor blocker

**Table 5:** Drugs requiring little or no dose adjustment.

| ***Drugs with alternative elimination pathways*** | ***Drugs with high therapeutic to toxic range*** |
|---|---|
| Amiodarone | Penicillins |
| Chloramphenicol/Linezolid/ Clindamycin/Doxycycline | Haloperidol |
| Ceftriaxone and cefoperazone | Cefuroxime |
| Alprazolam | Cefotaxime |
| Metoprolol/Carvedilol | Lignocaine |
| Betamethasone/ Dexamethasone | |
| Chlorpheniramine | |
| Haloperidol | |
| Rifampicin | |
| Ritonavir | |
| Heparin | |

**Box 2:** Key medications requiring dose adjustment or cessation in AKI.

- Analgesics morphine, meperidine, gabapentin, and pregabalin
- Antiepileptics lamotrigine
- *Antivirals:* Acyclovir, ganciclovir, and valganciclovir
- Antifungals fluconazole
- *Antimicrobials:* Almost all antimicrobials need dose adjustment in AKI with important exceptions like azithromycin, ceftriaxone, linezolid, nafcillin, doxycycline, and rifampin
- Diabetic agents sulfonylureas, metformin
- Allopurinol
- Baclofen
- Colchicine
- Digoxin
- Lithium
- Low-molecular-weight heparin
- NOACs

(AKI: acute kidney injury; NOACs: Novel oral anticoagulants)

cannot be used when the creatinine concentration is not in the steady state as in AKI. In severe AKI where the patient is oligoanuric, it is assumed that the GFR would be <10 mL/min when urine output is minimal (Table 5 and Box 2).

## RADIOCONTRAST-INDUCED NEPHROPATHY (RCIN)

It occurs in less than 1% in patients with normal renal function *but* increases significantly with renal insufficiency *though* dialysis is rarely needed for its treatment. Various risk factors can predispose to RCIN (Table 6).

### Clinical Characteristics

The onset of AKI occurs 24–48 hours after exposure to contrast media. It lasts for a duration of 5–7 days. It is a nonoliguric type of AKI in majority of cases. The urinary sediment may contain the "muddy-brown" pigmented casts and renal tubular cells typical of ATN or may be quite bland. There is a low fractional excretion of sodium in this condition.

**Table 6:** Risk Factors for radiocontrast-induced nephropathy (RCIN).

| ***Patient factors*** | ***Contrast related*** |
|---|---|
| Elderly | High osmolar contrast |
| Dehydration | Ionic contrast |
| Underlying CKD | High viscosity |
| Diabetes mellitus | Large volume |
| Urgent procedure | |
| Multiple myeloma | |
| CHF (LVEF <40%) | |
| Hypertension | |
| Low hematocrit | |
| Intra-aortic balloon pump | |

(CKD: chronic kidney disease; CHF: congestive heart failure; LVEF: left ventricular ejection fraction)

### Prophylactic Strategies

- Use intravenous (IV) contrast only when necessary.
- Hydration with normal saline (1–1.5 mL/kg/hr) 6–12 hours before and after the procedure is the only treatment shown to reduce RCIN.

- Use Low or iso-osmolar (nonionic) contrast media.
- Minimize contrast volume.
- N-acetylcysteine—600–1,200 mg bid for two doses before and two doses after the procedure may be used.

## SEPSIS AND ACUTE KIDNEY INJURY

Acute kidney injury occurs in 19% of patients with sepsis, 23% with severe sepsis, and in 51% with septic shock when blood cultures are positive. The combination of AKI and sepsis is associated with a 70% mortality rate, as compared to a mortality rate of 45% among patients with AKI alone. Nitric oxide synthases, cytokines, chemokines, and adhesion molecules play a role in AKI when it is associated with sepsis. The use of early goal-directed therapy in sepsis appears to reduce mortality rates among patients with AKI as described above.

## SUMMARY AND CONCLUSION

Acute kidney injury remains a ubiquitous medical condition and is associated with a high rate of mortality. Recent advances in defining and understanding AKI promise to help clinicians better diagnose and treat patients with this burdensome syndrome. Future research into the mechanisms and pathophysiology of AKI will elucidate the pathways of this complex disease process. As the clinical management of AKI remains largely supportive, the importance of primary disease prevention is clear.

## ACKNOWLEDGMENTS

1. Dr Valentine Lobo, Consultant Nephrologist, KEM Hospital, Pune.
2. Art work: Dr Milan C Patel, Registrar IDCCM, Jehangir Hospital, Pune.

## BIBLIOGRAPHY

1. Bellomo R, Kellum JA, Ronco C. Acute kidney injury. Lancet. 2012;380:756-66.
2. Bhadade R, De'Souza R, Harde MJ, et al. A prospective study of acute kidney injury according to KDIGO definition and its mortality predictors. J Assoc Physicians India. 2016;64(12):22-28.
3. Dellinger R Phillip, Vincent .Jean Louis, Silva et al. Surviving sepsis in developing countries. Critical Care Med. 2008;36(8):2487-88.
4. Kellum JA, Bellomo R, Ronco C. The concept of acute kidney injury and the RIFLE criteria. Contrib Nephrol. 2007;156:10-6.
5. Kher V, Srisawat N. Prevention and therapy of acute kidney Injury in the developing world. Kidney Int Rep. 2017;2(4):544-58.
6. Moore PK, Hsu RK, Kathleen D, et al. Management of acute kidney injury: Core Curriculum. Am J Kidney Dis. 2018;72(1):136-48.
7. Rhodes Andrew, et al. Surviving, Sepsis Campaign: International Guidelines Management of Sepsis and Septic Shock. Critical care Medicine. 2017;45(3):486-522.
8. Ricci Z, Cruz D, Ronco C. The RIFLE criteria and mortality in acute kidney injury: A systematic review. Kidney Int. 2008 Mar;73(5):538-46.
9. Rodrigues FB, Bruetto RG, Torres US, et al. Incidence and mortality of acute kidney injury after myocardial infarction: a comparison between KDIGO and RIFLE criteria. PLoS One. 2013:23;8(7):e69998.

CHAPTER 2

# Biomarkers in Acute Kidney Injury

*Siddhesh Dhaygude*

## INTRODUCTION

Acute kidney injury (AKI) represents acute decline in kidney function which is associated with increased morbidity, mortality, cost of therapy, and hospital stay. AKI can be the cause of late decline of kidney function in future. There are many genes, proteins, and enzymes which are up regulated during AKI out of which some of them can be used for the earlier diagnosis of AKI earlier or prediction of outcome. This may in future help to choose various therapeutic options and interventions.

## DEFINITION OF ACUTE KIDNEY INJURY

The KDIGO (Kidney Disease Improving Global Outcome) clinical practice guidelines define AKI as any of the following:

- Increase in serum creatinine by >0.3 mg/dL within 48 hours.
- Increase in serum creatinine to >1.5 times baseline which is known to or presumed to have occurred in the prior 7 days.
- Urine volume <0.5 mL/kg/hr for 6 hours.

The above definition is proposed by merging Risk, Injury, Failure, Loss of kidney function, and End-stage kidney disease (RIFLE) scheme of classification and Acute Kidney Injury Network (AKIN) classification.

As we know, AKI spectrum is changing in the developing world. Paradigm is shifting from infectious diseases, dehydration, and toxin-induced AKI to intensive care unit (ICU)-acquired AKI. This is due to better availability of healthcare facilities and early treatment initiation. As in the developed world, AKI in developing world is also seen more in ICU admitted patients with multiorgan dysfunction, elderly population, with multiple comorbidities.

## CONVENTIONAL MARKERS FOR AKI

As per RIFLE, AKIN, and KDIGO, the diagnosis world over is made based on:

- Serum creatinine/blood urea nitrogen (BUN)

- Urine output (UOP)
- Physical examination and clinical judgment.

However there are some pitfalls of using serum creatinine, which is considered up till now gold standard in diagnosis of AKI.

- It is slow to rise after kidney injury
- There can be variation in creatinine production due to diet, muscle mass, dilution, etc.
- Variation in creatinine secretion by tubules in initial period of AKI
- Extra renal creatinine excretion like gut
- Issues with measurement methodology and standardization.

Due to these reasons, search for newer molecules is going on with the intention to diagnose AKI earlier so that we can intervene if possible early to prevent progression, early withdrawal of offending drugs and prognostication of the disease.

## BIOMARKER

National Institute of Health (NIH) has described biomarker as characteristic that is objectively evaluated and is used to evaluate:

- Biological process
- Pathological process
- Response to therapeutic intervention.

### Types of Biomarkers[1,2]

For the ease of understanding, biomarkers are divided into four major categories (Table 1).

During last few years, various molecules have been identified or evaluated which either are derived from injured kidneys or reflect alteration in kidney function. These can be released from kidneys or upregulated due to altered kidney function. They can be from nonrenal tissues. These biomarkers can be used to differentiate nature, severity of AKI, and site of injury depending on their specificity (Table 2).

**Table 1:** Types of biomarkers.

| *Sr. No.* | *Types of biomarker* | *Examples* |
|---|---|---|
| 1 | Functional biomarker | Serum creatinine, BUN, serum cystatin C |
| 2 | Upregulated proteins | NGAL, KIM-1, L-FABP, IL-18 |
| 3 | Low-molecular-weight proteins and cytokines | Urine cystatin C and urinary activin A |
| 4 | Enzymes | NAG, αGST, πGST, GGT, and alkaline phosphatase |

(BUN: blood urea nitrogen; NGAL: neutrophil gelatinase-associated lipocalin; KIM-1: kidney injury molecule-1; L-FABP: liver fatty acid-binding protein; IL-18: interleukin-18; NAG: N-acetyl-β-D-glucosaminidase; πGST: pi-glutathione S transferase; GGT: gamma-glutamyl transpeptidase)

**Table 2:** Site of injury.[3-6]

| *Sr. No.* | *Site of injury* | *Biomarker* |
|---|---|---|
| 1 | Glomerulus | Total protein, urinary cystatin C, β2 microglobulin, α1 microglobulin, and albumin |
| 2 | Proximal tubules | KIM1, clusterin, NGAL, GSTα, β2 microglobulin, NAG, osteopontin, urinary cystatin C, netrin 1, RBP, IL-18, HGF, Cyr 61, NHE-3, exosomal fetuin-A, L-FABP, and albumin |
| 3 | Distal tubules | Osteopontin, clusterin, GST μ/π, NGAL, H-FABP, calbindin D28 |
| 4 | Collecting duct | Calbindin D28 |
| 5 | Loop of Henle | Osteopontin, NHE-3 |

(GST: glutathione-S-transferase; HGF: hepatocyte growth factor; IL-18: interleukin-18; KIM 1: kidney injury molecule 1; L-FABP: liver-type fatty-acid-binding protein; NGAL: neutrophil gelatinase-associated lipocalin; NAG: N-acetyl-β-D-glucosaminidase; NHE-3: sodium/hydrogen exchanger isoform 3; RBP: retinol-binding protein)

## Characteristics of an Ideal Biomarker

An ideal biomarker should be:

- Highly sensitive and specific
- Rapid and reliable increase in response to kidney disease
- Good correlation with degree of renal injury
- Provide risk stratification and prognostic information
- Site specific to detect early kidney injury and identify pathologic changes in specific segments of renal tubules.
- Applicable across different races and age groups.
- Allow recognition of cause of kidney injury or diseases (e.g. ischemia, toxins, sepsis, etc.)
- Organ specific and allows differentiation among intrarenal, prerenal, and extrarenal cause of kidney injury.
- Noninvasive
- Identify duration of kidney injury (acute vs. chronic)
- Useful to monitor the response to therapeutic interventions
- Provide information on the risk of complications from comorbid conditions.

## Biomarkers in Acute Kidney Injury[1,2]

### *Glomerular*

- *Serum creatinine*: It is a product of creatine and phosphocreatine which are involved in energy metabolism of skeletal muscles. It is freely filtered by glomerulus but to a less degree (10–30%) secreted by the proximal tubules. Its production varies greatly with age, gender, muscle mass, diet, and certain disease states, e.g. rhabdomyolysis. It is not site specific and cannot differentiate etiology like prerenal, intrinsic renal or post renal injury of sites like glomerulus, tubules proximal vs distal. Static measurement of serum creatinine does not reflect the real time changes in glomerular filtration rate (GFR). Creatinine secretion can be interfered by drugs like trimethoprim. Creatinine clearance may overestimate kidney function due to secretion.

- *Blood urea nitrogen:* It is product of protein metabolism and freely filtered at glomerulus. 30–70% can be reabsorbed. Its production is affected by endogenous protein catabolism, fluid intake, liver disease, etc. In the presence of renal disease urea clearance may underestimate kidney function due to reabsorption.
- *Cystatin C (CyC)*: It is a low-molecular-weight protein that is member of cysteine protease inhibitors superfamily. It is freely filtered at glomerulus and not reabsorbed. It is metabolized in tubules completely hence normally not detected in urine. Its production presumably thought to be constant and not affected by diet. Though initially it was thought that levels of cystatin C are not affected by age, gender or muscle mass, now it has been shown that higher levels of serum cystatin C are shown to be associated with male gender, high lean body mass, diabetes, hyper- and hypothyroidism, and age.

  Any impairment of reabsorption in proximal tubules can lead to marked increase in urinary levels of cystatin C. Its half-life is 2 hours so a better marker for detecting changes in GFR. It is measured by nephelometric assay.

  Various studies have been done to compare the utility of cystatin C to serum creatinine. In patients with cardiovascular disease, cystatin C levels showed stronger risk relationship with mortality than serum creatinine. In general population also few studies have shown higher levels of serum cystatin C are associated with poor cardiovascular outcomes in elderly.

  In a study which included 85 critically ill patients, 50% rise in serum cystatin C levels were noted a day or two earlier compared to serum creatinine with area under curve 0.97 and 0.82 respectively. Thus serum cystatin was superior to serum creatinine in detection of AKI RIFLE stage I and F. Also it showed good correlation with requirement of renal replacement therapy (RRT) in due course. In various settings like postcontrast administration, emergency department admissions with multiorgan dysfunction syndrome (MODS), serum cystatin C can predict development of AKI early but serial assessment does not show its superiority over serum creatinine data in various studies.

  In few studies, urinary cystatin C was found to be better marker than serum cystatin C in predicting AKI and morbidity. Also along with $\alpha 1$ microglobulin it has been shown to predict worse outcome in acute tubular necrosis (ATN). However need to have stronger data on this.

  However at present there is no strong data which shows that knowledge of serum cystatin C would alter clinical practice compared with data on creatinine at present.
- *Beta trace proteins (BTPs)*: It is a small molecular weight protein also called prostaglandin D synthase. It belongs to lipocalin protein family which is involved in binding and transport of small hydrophobic ligands. Primarily produced in cerebrospinal fluid. It is primarily eliminated by glomerular filtration. BTP has been studied mainly in ICU patients and renal transplant patients. Its levels are not affected by age or race. However, data has not been validated in larger studies and lack of a widespread standard assay availability limits its use in clinical practice.

## Tubular Injury Markers[1,2,6]

After tubular injury, three types of potential biomarkers are considered (Table 3).

**Table 3:** Tubular injury markers.

| | |
|---|---|
| Tubular injury | Tubular proteins getting regulated after injury |
| | Tubular proteins released after cell injury |
| | Cytokines and other markers released by inflammatory cells |

1. *Kidney injury molecule-1 (KIM-1)*: It was first described in 1998. Also called T cell immunoglobulin and mucin domains containing protein 1 (TIM-1), hepatitis A virus cellular receptor 1 (HAVCR 1) or cochlear injury molecule 1 (CIM 1).

   It is type 1 transmembrane glycoprotein which is significantly expressed in kidneys, specifically in proximal tubule after ischemic injury. It is not expressed in normal kidneys. Its presumptive role is in regeneration process and removal of dead cells by phagocytosis. Kidney is the only source of KIM-1.
   - Higher expression in proximal convoluted tubular cells of the kidney than any other cells of kidney or any other organ.
   - Structurally KIM-1 has single transmembrane domain which undergoes proximal cleavage and release of soluble ectodomain of KIM-1 in urine which is detected in setting of tubular injury. It is expressed in proximal tubular epithelial cells until complete recovery occurs.
   - Not detected in healthy kidneys.

   Many small studies have demonstrated utility of KIM-1. It has been shown to rise within 12 hours of kidney injury, much earlier than appearance of granular casts in urine. Higher levels of KIM-1 in urine are indicative of adverse outcomes in established AKI in the form of death or need for RRT. In patients of renal transplant, increased urinary levels of KIM-1 are associated with adverse graft outcomes.

   In the patients of postcardiac surgery, KIM-1 predicted AKI at 12 hours postoperative. In the meta-analysis done by Shao X et al. 11 studies were included and 2,979 patients studied. This showed KIM-1 led to early diagnosis of AKI with sensitivity of 74% and specificity of 86%. Initially KIM-1 was detected by enzyme-linked immunosorbent assay (ELISA) and then microbeads assay. But now urinary dipstick is also available which allows use at the point of care.
2. *Neutrophil gelatinase-associated lipocalin (NGAL)*: It is 25 kDa protein with 178 amino acids. It is a glycoprotein bound to matrix metalloproteinase-9 in human neutrophils. It is expressed in salivary glands, prostate, uterus, trachea, lung, stomach, and kidney. Its expression is markedly induced in injured epithelial cells. It is a potent epithelial cell growth inducer. It protects cells from ischemic injury. It is measured by ELISA.

   Its utility in diagnosing AKI has been mainly studied in pediatric populations undergoing cardiopulmonary bypass, where exact time of insult is known. In this population, a study by Mishra et al. has shown 100% sensitivity and 98% specificity in diagnosing AKI. Rise in levels have been shown to occur within 2 hours of surgery. In other smaller studies in adult patients undergoing cardiac surgery urinary NGAL was found to be elevated at 1 hour postsurgery in whom AKI was present. In a small study in pediatric and adult patients undergoing kidney transplant, higher urinary NGAL levels correlated with need for RRT and delayed allograft function. In another study from India in patients getting admitted in ICU, urinary NGAL at the time of admission of ICU exhibited good predictive ability of AKI, however, sensitivity was low. Up till now urinary NAGL has been studied in various AKI setting but results are variable hence needs larger studies to conclude its utility.[7]

3. *Interleukin-18 (IL-18)*: It is 18 kDa proinflammatory cytokine produced from renal tubular cells and macrophages. It is involved in mediating inflammatory process during ischemic, sepsis-induced or nephrotoxic AKI. It recruits neutrophils during inflammatory process; hence its levels are increased in tubular injury. It is measured by ELISA and microbead assay.

   In study of renal allograft recipients, elevated levels of IL-18 on day 0 were shown to predict delayed allograft function. In another study among 138 patients of acute respiratory distress syndrome (ARDS) levels of urinary IL-18 increased 24 hours prior to rise in serum creatinine level. It was also shown to predict mortality in this group. In critically ill patients, elevated levels of IL-18 have been shown as an independent predictor of mortality.

   Overall IL-18 is shown to be more specific for ischemic acute tubular injury. Its measurement may also be influenced by variables such as endotoxemia, immunologic injury, and cisplatin toxicity. IL-18 levels are also increased in conditions like inflammatory arthritis, inflammatory bowel disease, and systemic lupus erythematosus.

4. *α1 microglobulin*: It is a glycoprotein of 30 kDa from lipocalin superfamily which is synthesized in liver. It is freely filtered at glomerulus and completely reabsorbed and catabolized by normal proximal tubule. Hence elevated levels of α1 microglobulin indicate proximal tubular injury. It is measured by immune nephelometric assay or ELISA. It is more stable over pH range in urine compared to β2 microglobulin.

   In small study of 73 patients in whom 26 patients required RRT, cystatin C and α1 microglobulin had highest ability to predict the need for RRT. However, more studies are needed to accept this as reliable biomarker.

5. *β2 microglobulin*: It is 11.8 kDa protein from light chain of major histocompatibility complex class I which is present on cell surface of all nucleated cells. It is excreted by glomerular filtration and reabsorbed completely and catabolized by normal proximal tubule in human. It is measured by nephelometric assay. It is unstable at room temperature especially when urine pH is less than 5.5.

6. *Liver fatty acid-binding protein (L-FABP)*: These are small (15 kDg) cytoplasmic proteins which are abundantly expressed in tissues which have active fatty acid metabolism. These proteins facilitate long-chain fatty acid transport, regulate gene expression, and reduce oxidative stress. Normally these proteins are not detected in urine as megalin-mediated endocytosis completely absorbs L-FABP when there is ischemic kidney injury, this endocytosis mechanism is hampered and L-FABP appears in urine. Few small studies have studied this molecule in the setting of pediatric and adult cardiac surgery patients and kidney transplant which has shown to have correlation with development of AKI and need for RRT. However, larger studies are needed to confirm utility of this molecule.

7. *Netrin-1*: It is 50–75 kDa laminin-like protein which acts as chemotropic factor. It is under investigations as biomarker in AKI in animal models. Small human study in postcardiac surgery patient has shown correlation between rising urinary netrin-1 with severity of AKI and length of hospital stay.

8. *Insulin-like growth factor-binding protein (IGFBP) and tissue inhibitor of metalloproteinases 2 (TIMP2):*[8] Sepsis- and ischemia-induced tubular injuries are associated with regulation of various phases of cell cycles. Urinary IGFBP and TIMP2 are the two biomarkers identified which regulate cell cycle either by autocrine or paracrine manner and arrest cell cycle in G1 phase. In discovery (n = 522) and Sapphire study (n = 744), primary end point was KDIGO stage 2 or 3 AKI, in patients of sepsis or postsurgery. Both of the above biomarkers have been proved to be superior over the conventional biomarkers and clinical parameters like azotemia and oliguria. In addition, IGFBP and TIMP2 were helpful in identifying patient at risk of death or dialysis.

   Commercial kit to identify both of above biomarkers is under study and has got approval by US Food and Drug Administration in 2014 (NephroCheck™) though its appropriate timing of use and interpretation of results needs further validation. Commercial kits soon will be available in India.

   *Other under investigations biomarkers are* osteopontin, sodium-hydrogen exchanger isoform 3, clusterin, cysteine-rich protein, etc.

### *Tubular Enzymes*

- *N-acetyl-β-D-glucosaminidase (NAG)*: It is a lysosomal enzyme (>130 kDa) which is present in renal tubules. Because it has larger molecular weight, it cannot be filtered at glomerulus, hence when the levels are elevated, it comes from renal tubules. It excretion into urine correlates with lysosomal activity. It is more stable than other urinary enzymes. It is measured by colorimetry.

  In investigational studies, NAG level increases and precede creatinine level by 12 hours to 4 days. Elevated levels are found to predict outcome like death or need for dialysis in these patients. However larger studies are needed.

  Increased levels of urinary NAG have been reported to increased several nonrenal diseases like rheumatoid arthritis hyperthyroidism or conditions with increased lysosomal activity without cellular damage. Because it is sensitivity but less specific, clinical utility is limited as biomarker.
- *Alpha glutathione S transferase and pi glutathione S transferase (α-GST and π-GST)*: Both enzymes are from multigene family of detoxification enzymes; present in many organs including kidneys. These are distributed throughout nephron. Normally these are absent in urine. After renal injury α-GST is observed in proximal tubules while πGST in distal. Their ability to diagnose AKI earlier than conventional markers and specificity yet to be studied on larger scale.
- *Gamma-glutamyl transpeptidase (GGT) and alkaline phosphatase (AP)*: Both are tubular brush border enzymes and are released in urine whenever there is significant damage to brush border enzymes. These are yet to be studied in larger studies.

## Probable Role of Biomarkers in Treatment of AKI[2,5,6]

Probable role of biomarkers are considered in early diagnosis of AKI and may be in early probable initiation of RRT (Flowchart 1).

**Flowchart 1:** Role of biomarkers in AKI.

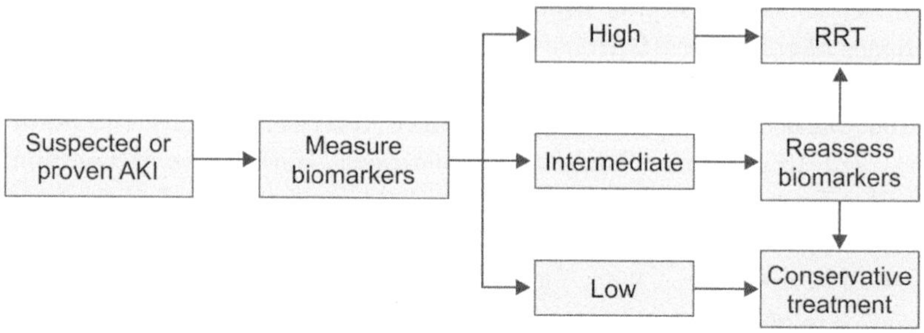


(AKI: acute kidney injury; RRT: renal replacement therapy)

## CONCEPT OF RENAL ANGINA (THE RENAL ANGINA INDEX)[9,10]

Concept of renal angina was first proposed by Goldstein and Chawala in critically ill pediatric population which refers to the state of kidney injury. Renal angina index (RAI) is a measure of renal angina (similar to cardiac angina in patients with acute coronary syndrome) easily calculated by using measures of kidney dysfunction and patient risk factors.

**RAI = AKI Risk score (Table 4) × AKI injury Score (Table 5) (Range 1–40)**

It has been postulated that use of renal angina index may help clinician to use biomarkers appropriately to diagnose AKI early in those patients who are at risk of developing the same. Otherwise estimation of various biomarkers can be false positive and may overdiagnose AKI. For example, Trop I may be false positive but in those patients having clinical symptoms and risk factors it is very helpful in diagnosis of acute coronary syndrome. Similarly RAI >8 and detection of biomarkers may help us to diagnose and manage AKI more efficiently. This index though first proposed in pediatric population now is being studied in the adult population also, for its utility.

## FUTURE DIRECTIONS

Keeping aside limitations of studies on various biomarkers, there are positive aspects of serum and urinary biomarkers. Urinary IL-18, KIM-1, and NAG performed extremely well in evaluation of established AKI. Serum cystatin C, urine NGAL, IL-18 performed well for early diagnosis. NAG, KIM-1, and IL-18 performed well for mortality risk prediction in AKI. Combination of various biomarkers may be considered in diagnosis and treatment of AKI.

**Table 4:** Acute kidney injury risk.

| *Risk factor* | *Level of risk* | *Score* |
|---|---|---|
| ICU admission | Medium | 1 |
| History of organ transplantation (solid/bone marrow) | High | 3 |
| Vasopressor support or mechanical ventilation | Very high | 5 |

**Table 5:** Acute kidney injury.

| *Change in estimated creatinine clearance from baseline* | *Fluid overload %* | *Severity score* |
|---|---|---|
| <0 | 0–5 | 1 |
| 1–1.49 | 5–9.99 | 2 |
| 1.5–1.99 | 10–14.99 | 4 |
| >2 | >15 | 8 |

However at this point of time, considering present data on various biomarkers, none of the biomarkers have shown additional clear advantage over clinical decision process and conventional investigations. Hence clinical evaluation and conventional investigations still remain gold standard in diagnosis and management of AKI.

## REFERENCES

1. Hilde R H de Geus, Betjes MG, Bakker J. Biomarkers for the prediction of acute kidney injury: a narrative review on current status and future challenges. Clin Kidney J. 2012;5(2):102-8.
2. Cia-Mei-Zheng, Min-Tser Liao, Mei-Yu Lin, et al. Biomarkers in acute kidney injury. Open J Nephrol. 2013;3:51-60.
3. Westenfelder C. Earlier diagnosis of acute kidney injury awaits effective therapy. Kidney Int. 2011;79(11):1159-61.
4. Ostermann M, Philips BJ, Forni LG. Clinical review: Biomarkers of acute kidney injury: where are we now? Crit Care. 2012;16(5):237.
5. Lameier NH, Vanholder RC, Van Biesen WA. How to use biomarkers efficiently in acute kidney injury. Kidney Int. 2011;79(10):1047-50.
6. Murray PT, Mehta RL, Shaw A, et al. Potential use of biomarkers in acute kidney injury: report and summary of recommendations from the 10th Acute Dialysis Quality Initiative consensus conference. Kidney Int. 2014;85(3):513-21.
7. NM Nayak, S Madhumitha, RA Annigeri, et al. Clinical utility of urine neutrophil gelatinase-associated lipocalin measured at admission to predict outcomes in heterogeneous population in critically ill patients. Indian J Nephrol. 2016;26(2):119-24.
8. Kashani K, Al-Khafaji A, Ardiles T, et al. Discovery and Validation of cell cycle arrest biomarkers in human acute kidney injury. Crit Care. 2013;6:17(1):R25.
9. Stuart L. Goldstein Renal Angina Index to Predict Acute Kidney Injury. Are Adults Just Large Children? Kidney Int Rep. 2018; 3(3):516-8.
10. Menon S, Goldstein S, Motters T, et al. Urinary biomarker incorporation into the renal angina index early in intensive care unit admission optimizes acute kidney injury prediction in critically ill children: a prospective cohort study. Nephrol Dial Transplant. 2016;31(4):586-94.

CHAPTER 3

# Principles of Renal Replacement Therapy in Critical Care

*Valentine Lobo*

## INTRODUCTION

The spectrum of acute kidney injury (AKI) remains mixed with single organ involvement injury in community-acquired AKI to being part of multiorgan involvement in intensive care unit (ICU)-acquired AKI. While the incidence of AKI in the community is difficult to determine and varies widely across countries and even among hospitals in the same region, the incidence of hospital-acquired AKI has been pegged at around 38 per 1,000[1] discharges in two large studies in the United States. When sepsis is the primary diagnosis, a progressive increase in the incidence of AKI is seen with increasing severity, being 17% with sepsis, 23% with severe sepsis, and 51% with septic shock with positive blood cultures.[1] When sepsis and a requirement for dialysis coexist in a critically ill patient the mortality is believed to be between 23% and 79%.[1] A recent review has estimated the incidence of AKI in critically ill patients at 57% with a mortality of 27%.[2]

Figure 1 shows a schematic of the interrelation between septic shock, acute kidney injury, and the role of therapy (iatrogenic factors) in worsening end organ damage and outcomes. The clinician caring for such patients is forced to compromise between maintaining a minimum intravascular volume and mean arterial pressure required to ensure vital organ perfusion and avoid organ edema with its deleterious consequences. In recent years the role of organ cross talk in producing dysfunction of the lungs, heart, brain, liver, and intestine, by aberrant organ-organ communication in AKI has been shown to be a factor impacting the high mortality of this condition.[2]

What is unique about critically ill patients is that multiple indications for renal replacement therapy (RRT) may exist simultaneously and a balance may have to be created between providing biochemical correction of hyperkalemia, acidosis and uremia, fluid removal for pulmonary edema, and maintenance of blood pressure in a patient with increased extravascular volume, inotrope need, and increased permeability of capillaries and veins. Figure 2 shows the complex interplay between the metabolic abnormalities, electrolyte and acid-base derangements, and fluid overload in the altered physiology of AKI. The goals of AKI are to correct the metabolic derangements and fluid overload without producing worsening of organ dysfunction by hypotension and hypoperfusion.

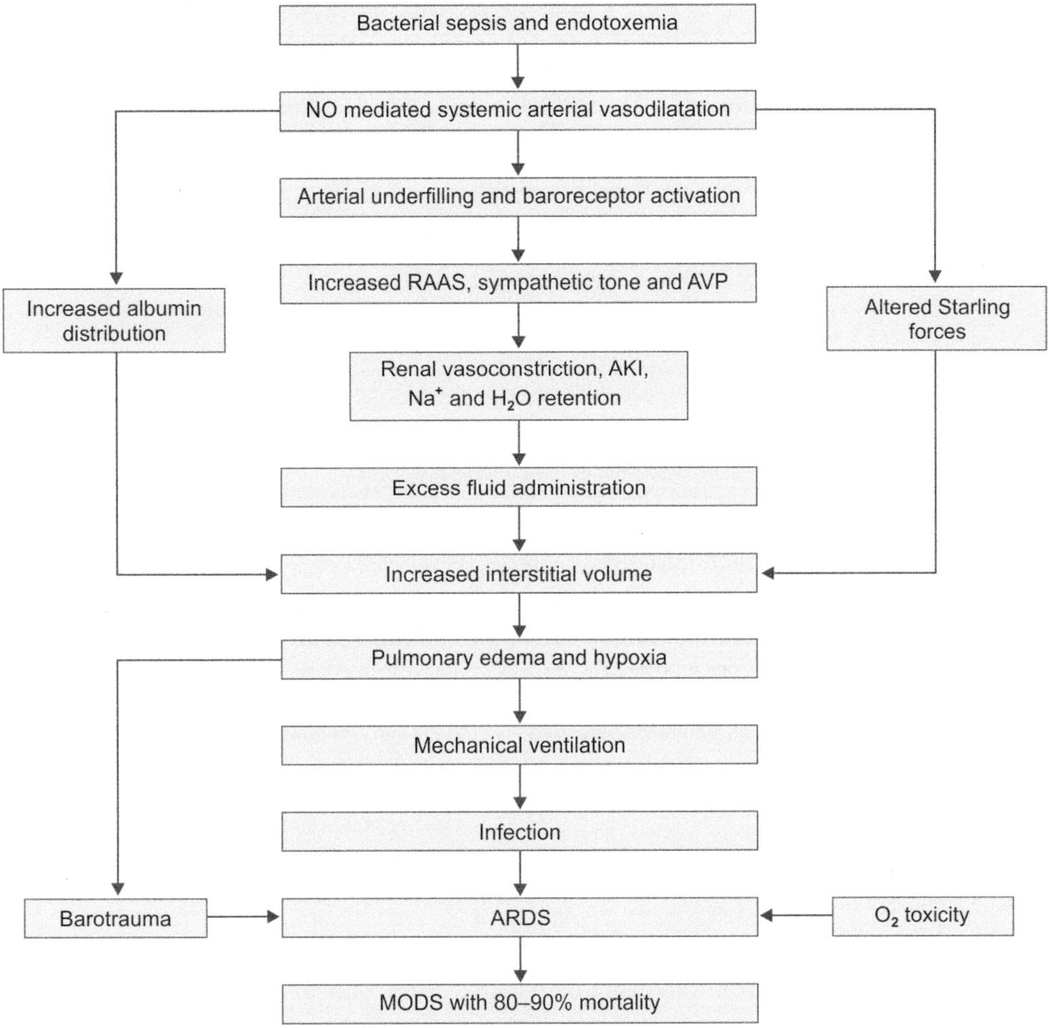


**Fig. 1:** Hemodynamic and organ function compromise in septic shock with AKI.

(AVP: arginine vasopressin; RAAS: renin-angiotensin-aldosterone system; AKI: acute kidney injury; ARDS: acute respiratory distress syndrome; MODS: multiorgan dysfunction syndrome)

It is now well established that in children with AKI a volume overload of 10% can worsen prognosis and an overload of 20% of body weight is associated with increased mortality.[3,4] A similar situation occurs in adults although the figures are less well established and the existing comorbidities act as confounders.

Table 1 shows the four primary processes used to clear solutes and fluid in RRT.[5]

1. *Diffusion*: This is governed by Ficks law, Diffusive Flux $J_d$ = DATdc/dx, where D is the diffusability coefficient, A the surface area and dc/dx the concentration gradient. Diffusion is typically bidirectional, with nitrogenous wastes, and hydrogen ions moving from blood to dialysate while calcium ions and buffers like bicarbonate moving in the reverse direction.

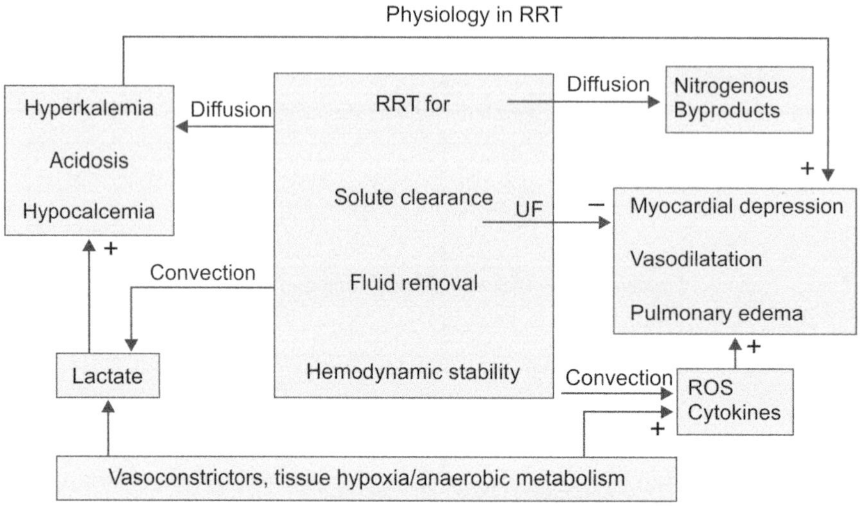


**Fig. 2:** Physiology in renal replacement therapy (RRT).
(ROS: reactive oxygen species; UF: ultrafiltration)

**Table 1:** Processes used to clear solutes and fluid in renal replacement therapy.

| | | |
|---|---|---|
| Diffusion | Solute moves from higher to lower concentration across a membrane | Small molecules like urea, creatinine, sodium, potassium, calcium, and bicarbonate |
| Ultrafiltration | Fluid driven through membrane pores by a pressure gradient | Water and other solvents |
| Convection | Solvent drags some dissolved solutes | Water soluble vitamins, beta 2 microglobulin, some cytokines, and chemokines |
| Adsorption | Molecules bind to specific membrane receptors | Endotoxin, cytokines, and inflammatory mediators |

Typically factors like the dialyzer surface area, blood flow, and counter current dialysate flow to maximize the concentration gradient increase the solute removal by diffusion. Small molecular weight solutes are cleared largely by diffusion.

2. *Ultrafiltration*: This refers to the movement or flux of fluid through a membrane caused by the application of a pressure. The pressure may be hydrostatic as in hemodialysis or continuous renal replacement therapy (CRRT) where the movement of fluid through a tube driven by a pump causes a lateral pressure on the walls of the tube, in this case the capillaries of the dialyzer or osmotic as occurs in peritoneal dialysis. By increasing the concentration of a less permeable solute in the dialysate the osmotic pressure of the dialysate solution is increased and causes the movement of water into the dialysate to achieve chemical osmotic equilibrium.
3. *Convection*: The movement of water carries with it dissolved solutes provided the pores which transport the water are permeable to the solute. The Hydraulic Permeability $Jc = Qf(Cb^*S) = Qf[Cb(1-\sigma)]$, where Qf is the fluid volume, Cb the concentration in the blood water, S is the sieving coefficient, which is = Cf/Cb and $\sigma$ is called the Staverman reflection coefficient. The sieving coefficient and the reflection coefficient have values between 0 and 1.

Smaller the molecular weight closer the sieving coefficient to 1 and the value approaches 0 as the molecular weight increases. The sieving coefficient for albumin of most conventional dialyzers and hemofilters is 0, though a few high cutoff membranes do permit the passage of proteins. The solute removal therefore by convection is proportional to the volume of ultrafiltrate removed and this offers a large capacity for solute removal as the treatment time increases.

4. *Adsorption*: This is the binding to specific receptors on the dialyzer membrane of certain solutes. The capacity for removal depends on the number of binding sites, their affinity for the solute, and their saturation with time.

Traditionally the patient's blood is spoken of as being cleared of a solute, a theoretical concept that presupposes a certain volume of blood being made free of the solute per unit time by a pass through the dialyzer. Individual solutes are cleared predominantly by diffusion, convection, adsorption or a variable combination of all three. Percentage of effective convective transport greater than 20% of the total processed blood is seen in hemofiltration or hemodiafiltration procedures, while the total clearance is the sum of all three.

The various renal replacement modalities that make use of these principles need to provide a predefined reduction in metabolic solute load, fluid removal, and correction of conditions like metabolic acidosis by providing a suitable buffer and most importantly they need to do this without worsening the fragile hemodynamic status of the ICU patient with AKI.

Table 2 provides a comparison of the two most widely used modalities of RRT utilized in ICUs the world over. While each of these have their relative advantages and disadvantages, typically costs, availability of trained personnel and material will often be the driving force for a particular treatment. With studies failing to provide proof of a survival advantage for either method, individual units may actually obtain the best results in terms of patient safety by adhering to that method of RRT with which the staff is most familiar.

Since the late 1990s a hybrid modality of therapy, variably called slow extended daily dialysis, sustained low-efficiency dialysis (SLED) or prolonged intermittent RRT, has gained increasing

**Table 2:** Comparison of continuous and intermittent renal replacement therapies.

| *Intermittent HD* | *Continuous renal replacement* |
|---|---|
| More time available for diagnostic and therapeutic procedures | Independent free standing easily operable machines |
| Lower risk of bleeding | Prolonged gradual eventual superior control of solutes and fluid |
| Rapid control of hyperkalemia and acidosis | Adequate nutrition possible |
| Less expensive and labour intensive | ? Cytokine removal |
| Specific infrastructure required | Better hemodynamic stability |
| Periodic solute control with risk of dysequilibrium | Higher risk of systemic bleeding |
| More frequent hypotensive episodes | Prolonged immobilization |
| | Much higher costs |
| | Frequent treatment interruptions |

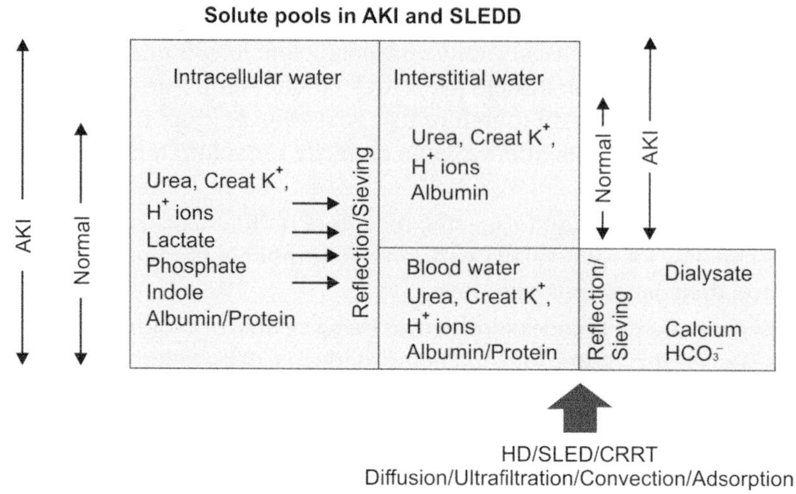


**Fig. 3:** Solute distribution and clearance in renal replacement therapy.

(AKI: acute kidney injury; CRRT: continuous renal replacement therapy; HD: hemodialysis; SLED: sustained low-efficiency dialysis; SLEDD: sustained low-efficiency daily dialysis)

acceptance the world over. This therapy is usually carried out for durations from 6 hours to 24 hours on conventional hemodialysis machines with appropriate modifications to blood flow, dialysate flow, and ultrafiltration rate (See the chapter on SLED for details).

The behavior of solutes during these various therapies is illustrated in Figure 3. It is obvious that a solute rebound occurs with intermittent therapies and not with continuous therapies and that the magnitude of the rebound is proportional to the interdialytic interval. This is caused by the fact that the dialyzer interfaces only with the blood water and solute and fluid exchange occurs only between these two pools. The two remaining pools, the interstitial and the intracellular water, are then cleared by their equilibration with the blood water (Fig. 4). The rate of solute equilibrium in comparison with dialyzer clearance determines the solute rebound and is also responsible for the phenomenon of dialysis disequilibrium. When a large drop in the concentration of a solute in the blood occurs, the osmolality of the blood water decreases, but because of the blood-brain barrier the brain cells remain hyperosmolar and water is transported intracellularly leading to brain swelling, increased intracranial pressure, and disequilibrium. The drop in serum osmolality also retards vascular refilling which is already impaired by increased capillary permeability and low albumin in critically ill patients. A lower clearance rate which preserves plasma osmolality and promotes refilling will therefore reduce the risks of hypotension and this is indeed the aim of both CRRT and SLED. While the exact rate of vascular refilling in the critically ill patient is unknown, stable chronic kidney disease (CKD) patients were shown to tolerate a fluid removal rate of 10–12 mL/kg/hr,[6,7] so a rate of around 50% or less than this should probably be targeted in the absence of studies providing any information. A compromise may often have to be made between providing adequate ultrafiltration to prevent and treat pulmonary edema. The ideal ultrafiltration rate has not been established in AKI but may be expected to be much lower than that shown in CKD patients in the Hemodialysis (HEMO) study above, given

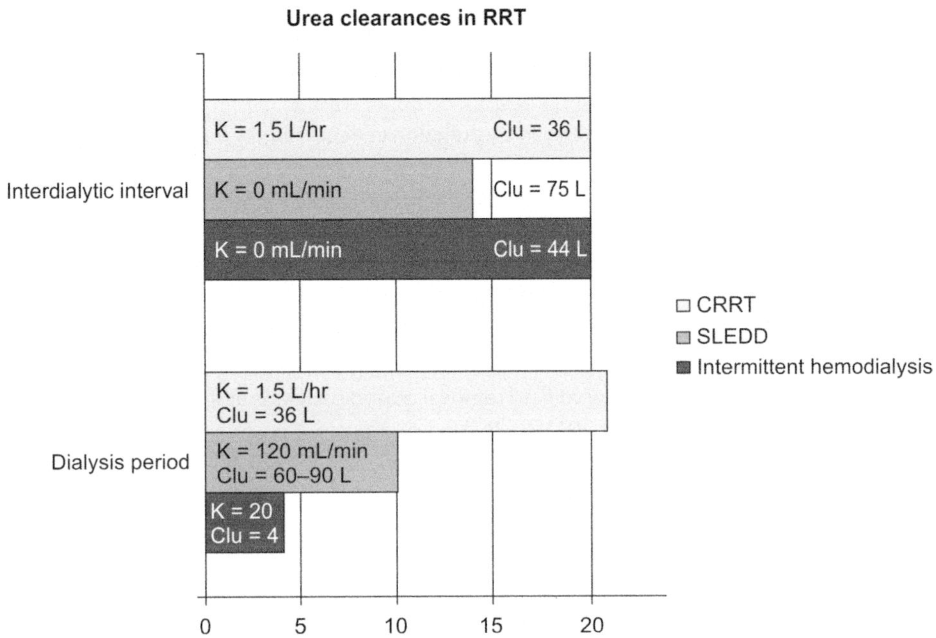


**Fig. 4:** Effects of dialytic and interdialytic time on clearance.
(CRRT: continuous renal replacement therapy; SLEDD: sustained low-efficiency daily dialysis; Clu: urea clearance)
*(For color version, see Plate 1)*

**Box 1:** Aims of renal replacement therapy (RRT).

- Define the primary goal of RRT daily to individualize prescription
  - Fluid removal
  - Acid/base control
  - Small solute clearance
- Maximize delivered vs. prescribed RRT ratio by using a high functioning dialysis vascular access
- Anticoagulation—primum non nocere
- Review appropriateness medication dosing daily, especially antimicrobial agents.
- Ensure appropriate nutrition support for continuous renal replacement therapy (CRRT)—augmented protein intake recommended
- Avoid RRT-related complications
- Severe hypophosphatemia (i.e. <2.0 mEq/L)
- Frequent CRRT circuit failures/increased blood transfusion needs
- Minimize therapy errors

that CKD patients are traditionally hypertensive and AKI ICU patients require vasopressor agents to maintain their blood pressure. A pediatric multicenter retrospective study showed an ultrafiltration rate of 9 mL/kg/hr to be safe, in most patients it will usually need to be lower.

The aims of RRT can be summarized in the Box 1.

As seen above the processes and procedures listed above may be utilized to deliver the goals listed here. Subsequent chapters will deal with the safety of anticoagulation, avoiding complications, and adjusting drug dosing during RRT.

## REFERENCES

1. Himmelfarb J, Ikizler TA. Acute kidney injury: changing lexicography, definitions, and epidemiology Kidney Int. 2007;71:971-6.
2. Lee SA, Cozzi M, Bush EL, et al. Distant Organ Dysfunction in Acute Kidney Injury: A Review. Am J Kidney Dis. 2018;72(6):846-56.
3. Li Y, Wang J, Bai Z, et al. Early fluid overload is associated with acute kidney injury and PICU mortality in critically ill children. Eur J Pediatr. 2016;175(1):39-48.
4. Diaz F, Benfield M, Brown L, et al. Fluid overload and outcomes in critically ill children: A single center prospective cohort study. J Crit Care. 2017;39:209-13.
5. Forni LG, Hilton PJ. Continuous hemofiltration in the treatment of acute renal failure. N Engl J Med. 1997;336:1303-9.
6. Flythe JE, Kimmel SE, Brunelli SM. Rapid fluid removal during dialysis is associated with cardiovascular morbidity and mortality. Kidney Int. 2011;79(2):250-7.
7. Sethi SK, Sinha R, Jha R, et al. Feasibility of sustained low efficiency dialysis in critically sick pediatric patients: A multicentric retrospective study. Hemodial Int. 2018;22(2):228-34.

CHAPTER 4

# Renal Replacement Therapy: Nomenclature and Terminology

*Sachin S Soni, Shriganesh R Barnela, Sonali S Saboo, Unmesh V Takalkar, Suresh H Saboo*

## INTRODUCTION

The term renal replacement therapy (RRT), when used for patients suffering from chronic kidney disease (CKD), encompasses a wide spectrum of therapies which include hemodialysis, peritoneal dialysis, and kidney transplantation. However, when discussed in relation to critically ill patients, RRT is a broad term used for various types extracorporeal therapies utilized to manage acute kidney injury (AKI) and other organ dysfunction syndromes in intensive care units (ICUs). In this chapter, we will discuss the later.

We will discuss RRT nomenclature and terminology under two major heads—dialysis process related and therapy type (Table 1). We will also briefly discuss terminologies related to other "nonrenal" extracorporeal therapies in ICUs used as multiorgan support therapies (MOST).

## PROCESS RELATED

Process of dialysis is based on three basic physiological principles—diffusion, convection, and osmosis.

**Table 1:** Renal replacement therapy nomenclature.

| *Process* | *Therapy type* |
|---|---|
| 1. Diffusion | 1. Intermittent hemodialysis (IHD) |
| 2. Convection | 2. Sustained low-efficiency dialysis (SLED) |
| 3. Osmosis | 3. *Continuous renal replacement therapy (CRRT)*:<br>– Slow continuous ultrafiltration (SCUF)<br>– Continuous arteriovenous hemofiltration (CAVH)<br>– Continuous arteriovenous hemodialysis (CAVHD)<br>– Continuous venovenous hemofiltration (CVVH)<br>– Continuous venovenous hemodialysis (CVVHD)<br>– Continuous venovenous hemodiafiltration (CVVHDF) |

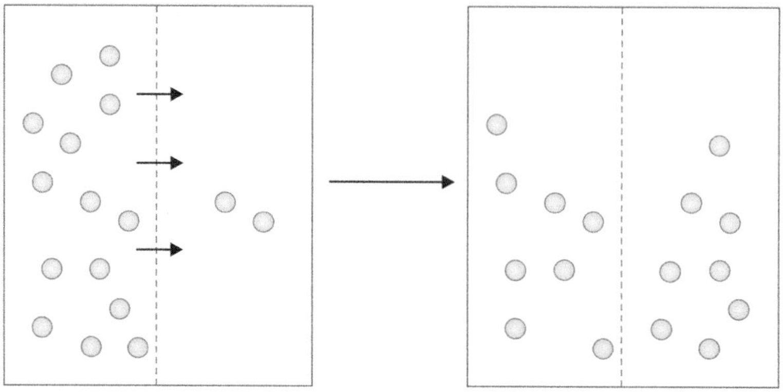

Movement of solutes form high to low concentration across a semipermeable membrane

**Fig. 1:** Diffusion. *(For color version, see Plate 2)*

## Diffusion

Diffusion is movement of solutes as a result of random molecular motions across a semipermeable membrane down its concentration gradient (Fig. 1). During hemodialysis most of the toxin removal is accomplished by diffusion. It is the best method for small solute clearance.

## Convection

Ultrafiltration (UF) is the process of water removal during dialysis with the help of by transmembrane pressure gradient. Water also drags some solutes along, contributing to solute clearance. This solvent drag during UF is known as convection. It contributes to middle molecule clearance.

## Osmosis

Osmosis is movement of water from low to high osmolar solution across a semipermeable membrane. This physiologic principle is utilized during peritoneal dialysis. Peritoneal cavity is filled with dialysis fluid with high osmolality which in turn helps in UF and removal of uremic toxins from the patient.

# THERAPY RELATED

## Intermittent Hemodialysis

Intermittent hemodialysis (IHD) is the most frequent form of RRT utilized in routine clinical practice. This therapy utilizes both diffusive and convective forms of clearances. It needs a large bore venous access. A typical IHD session runs for 3–4 hours with blood flow rate (Qb) of about 200–350 mL/min and dialysate flow rate (Qd) of 500 mL/min. UF rate depends on patient's hydration and hemodynamic status, but is generally around 500 mL/hr. In most cases, unfractionated heparin is utilized as anticoagulation to maintain patency of extracorporeal circuit.

## Continuous Renal Replacement Therapies

Continuous renal replacement therapy (CRRT) has emerged as a dialysis technique of choice in critically ill patients.[1] As the nomenclatures itself suggests, it is a continuous form of dialysis. It is being increasingly utilized in hemodynamically unstable patients who require ongoing, large-volume fluid administration, like multiple intravenous medications or parenteral nutrition.[2] Continuous arteriovenous hemofiltration (CAVH) and continuous arteriovenous hemodialysis (CAVHD) are described as early forms of CRRT. In this technique, a direct arterial access is utilized as blood pump to the extracorporeal circuit and blood is returned back using a separate venous access. With availability of sophisticated machines, such forms of CRRT are almost obsolete and will not be discussed any further in this chapter.

Currently, large bore double lumen venous access is utilized in all forms of CRRT. Anticoagulation protocols for CRRT include use of heparin, heparin free or regional citrate anticoagulation. CRRT can be provided in various forms depending on patient specific requirements, available resources, and staff skills.[3]

### *Slow Continuous Ultrafiltration*

Slow continuous ultrafiltration (SCUF) (Fig. 2) is used for patients with refractory fluid overload, with or without kidney disease. It is generally used for patients with refractory congestive cardiac failure. Its primary aim is to achieve safe and effective fluid removal to correct overload state. Solute removal is minimal.

### *Continuous Venovenous Hemofiltration*

Continuous venovenous hemofiltration (CVVH) (Fig. 3) uses convection as mode of solute removal. Its primary aim is to achieve high volume UF to be replaced in part or completely with appropriate replacement fluids. CVVH is designed to achieve both solute clearance and volume control. Replacement fluid can be infused before the hemofilter (predilution method), after the

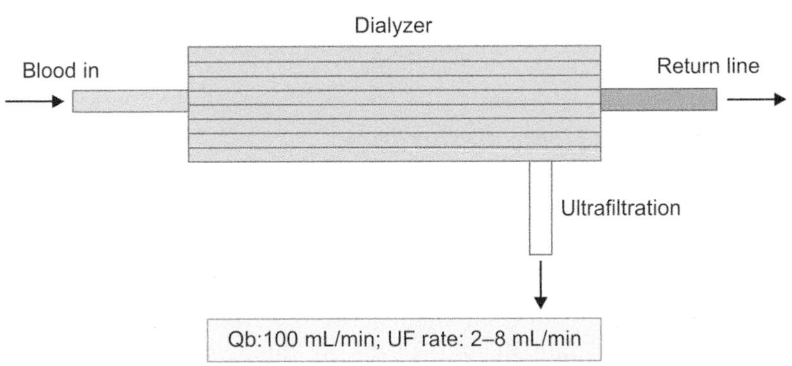


**Fig. 2:** Slow continuous ultrafiltration. *(For color version, see Plate 2)*

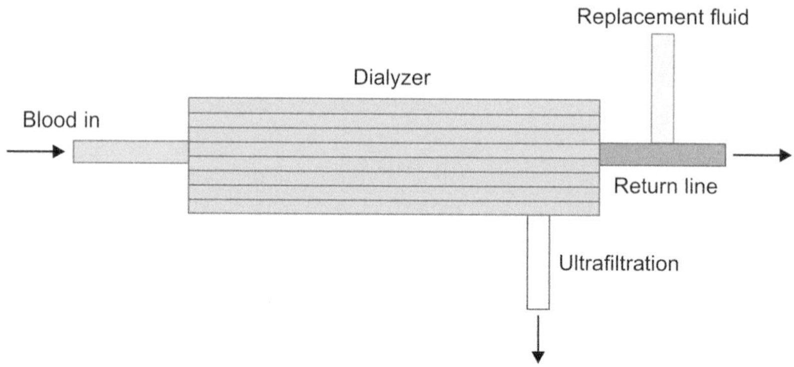


**Fig. 3:** Continuous venovenous hemofiltration.
(UF: ultrafiltration) *(For color version, see Plate 2)*

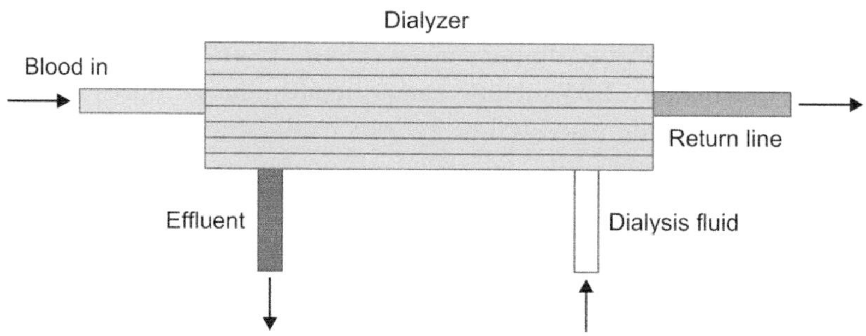


**Fig. 4:** Continuous venovenous hemodialysis. *(For color version, see Plate 3)*

hemofilter (postdilution method) or combination of both. A typical CVVH prescription includes Qb of 100–200 mL/min and UF rate of 600–1500 mL/hr.

## *Continuous Venovenous Hemodialysis*

Continuous venovenous hemodialysis (CVVHD) (Fig. 4) is a continuous form of hemodialysis performed at lower Qb. It uses diffusion as mode of solute removal. Dialysis fluid runs in counter current direction to blood to achieve slow diffusive clearance. A typical CVVH prescription includes Qb of 100–200 mL/min, UF rate of 100–250 mL/hr, and dialysate flow rate of 100–300 mL/min.

## *Continuous Venovenous Hemodiafiltration*

Continuous venovenous hemodiafiltration (CVVHDF) (Fig. 5) uses convection as mode of solute removal. Its primary aim is to achieve high volume UF to be replaced in part or completely with appropriate replacement fluids. CVVH is designed to achieve both solute clearance and volume control. Replacement fluid can be infused before the hemofilter (predilution method), after the hemofilter (postdilution method) or combination of both. A typical CVVH prescription includes Qb of 100–200 mL/min and UF rate of 600–1,500 mL/hr. Table 2 shows comparison of common CRRT subtypes with respect to infused fluids and method of solute clearance.

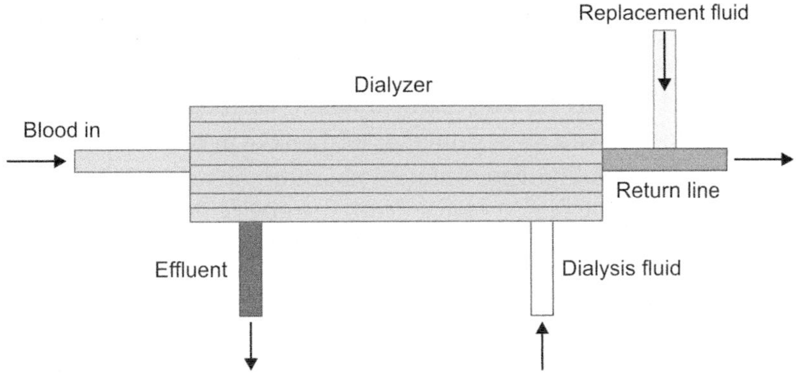


**Fig. 5:** Continuous venovenous hemodiafiltration. *(For color version, see Plate 3)*

**Table 2:** Comparison of various continuous renal replacement therapy subtypes.

| | *Fluids* | | *Method of solute clearance* | |
|---|---|---|---|---|
| *Modality* | *Dialysate* | *Replacement fluid* | *Diffusion* | *Convection* |
| SCUF | No | No | No | Minimal |
| CVVH | No | Yes | No | Yes |
| CVVHD | Yes | No | Yes | No |
| CVVHDF | Yes | Yes | Yes | Yes |

(SCUF: slow continuous ultrafiltration; CVVH: continuous venovenous hemofiltration; CVVHD: continuous venovenous hemodialysis; CVVHDF: continuous venovenous hemodiafiltration)

## Sustained Low-efficiency Dialysis

Sustained low-efficiency dialysis (SLED) is a hybrid treatment that provides RRT for an extended period of time, typically 6–10 hours, but is intermittent or discontinuous. SLED offers clearance through both diffusion and convection. These therapies attempt to utilize the advantages of slow therapies and minimize the disadvantages of continuous therapies. SLED offers efficient solute removal (similar to IHD) and delivers slower UF rate for hemodynamically unstable patients. Its shorter duration (compared to CRRT) offers other advantages like less anticoagulant exposure, lower costs, and decreased nurse workload.[4] It also liberates patient from machine for some hours to undergo other important diagnostic and interventional procedures if needed.

Hybrid therapies are also variably labeled as slow low-efficiency extended daily dialysis, accelerated venovenous hemofiltration (AVVH), prolonged intermittent RRT (PIRRT), extended dialysis (ED), extended daily dialysis (EDD), extended daily dialysis with filtration (EDDf), and go slow dialysis.

Sustained low-efficiency dialysis is usually performed using standard hemodialysis machine having ability to set lower dialysate flow rate (Qd). Normally, IHD machines are set to function at Qd of 500 mL/min. In SLED the desired Qd is around 100–300 mL/min. A typical SLED session runs for 6–8 hours with blood flow rate (Qb) of about 100–150 mL/min. UF rate depends on patients' hydration and hemodynamic status, and is generally around 100–250 mL/hr.

## OTHER EXTRACORPOREAL THERAPIES IN ICU

Many other extracorporeal therapies are utilized in the ICU for removal of variable toxins not cleared by conventional RRT techniques. In critically ill patients, initial impairment of one organ function is often followed by dysfunction or damage in other organs.[5] Main purpose of such therapies is to treat multiorgan dysfunction syndrome with MOST. Examples of such therapies are: therapeutic plasma exchange (TPE), extracorporeal membrane oxygenation therapy (ECMO), liver dialysis, and blood purification in sepsis

### Therapeutic Plasma Exchange

Therapeutic plasma exchange is a procedure in which the patient's blood is passed through an apheresis machine, where the filtered plasma is removed and discarded with reinfusion of replacement fluid such as plasma or albumin to the patient.[6] TPE is indicated in the treatment of many neurological renal and rheumatological diseases. Recent evidences suggest its role as an adjunctive therapy in sepsis and septic shock.

### Extracorporeal Membrane Oxygenation Therapy

Extracorporeal membrane oxygenation therapy is an extracorporeal technique of providing prolonged cardiac and respiratory support to patients with failing heart and lungs. The therapy aims to provide an adequate amount of gas exchange or perfusion to sustain life. ECMO is also known as extracorporeal life support.

### Liver Dialysis

Liver dialysis or artificial liver support devices are designed to remove toxins accumulated in patients with liver disease. Conventional RRT removes water-soluble toxins, however, liver dysfunction leads to accumulation of lipophilic and albumin bound toxins like bilirubin, bile acids, medium-chain fatty acids, nitric oxide, amino acid metabolites, and cytokines which are not removed by hemodialysis.[7] Albumin-rich dialysate is necessary for removal of such toxins. Currently three liver dialysis systems are in use—single pass albumin dialysis, molecular adsorbent recirculating system (MARS), and fractionated plasma separation and adsorption system (Prometheus, Fresenius Medical Care, Germany).

### Blood Purification in Sepsis

Sepsis is the primary cause of death in the ICU. Extracorporeal blood purification therapies have been proposed to improve outcomes for patients with sepsis. These therapies target removal of inflammatory mediators or bacterial toxins (or both) from the circulation to favorably modulate the host inflammatory response. Recent technological advances have greatly broadened the spectrum of available techniques for blood purification in sepsis.

### High-volume Hemofiltration

High-volume hemofiltration is a form of CRRT with target UF rate greater than 35 mL/kg/hr using high flux membranes. Beneficial effects of this technique are postulated to be related to removal of inflammatory cytokines during the early phase of sepsis which in turn can stop the inflammatory cascade, limit organ damage, and consequently decrease the incidence of multiorgan failure syndrome.[8]

### Continuous Plasma Filtration Coupled with Adsorption

Continuous plasma filtration coupled with adsorption is a two-step detoxification therapy. In first step, a plasma filter separates plasma from the blood which is then pumped over an adsorbent cartridge containing a resin with high affinity to many cytokines, mediators, and toxins. The purified plasma is then returned to the main circuit where blood is reconstituted. The plasma passes through the adsorbent cartridge with a lower velocity than the blood flow which allows more efficient removal of inflammatory mediators.[9]

### Hemoperfusion

Hemoperfusion involves placement of a sorbent cartridge in series with the filter in order to remove those toxins that are not removable by classic CRRT. The sorbent is placed in direct contact with blood and toxin removal characteristics of hemoperfusion are dependent on the types of sorbent used. Polymyxin (PMX)-hemoperfusion utilizes PMX B-coated fibers in a cartridge with high affinity for lipopolysaccharide which helps in removal of circulating endotoxin.[10]

The CytoSorb adsorber, which is approved for use in European market and also available in India, is composed of biocompatible porous polymer beads that act like tiny sponges to remove substances from whole blood based on pore capture and surface adsorption. This technique is also designed to reduce cytokine burden during sepsis.

## SUMMARY

Incidence of acute kidney injury in critically ill patients is steadily increasing. Development of AKI is associated with increased morbidity and mortality. Familiarity with various renal replacement modalities and associated terminologies is essential for all intensive care physicians.

## REFERENCES

1. Ronco C, Bellomo R. Continuous renal replacement therapy: evolution in technology and current nomenclature. Kidney Int Suppl. 1998;66:S160-4.
2. Ronco C, Bellomo R. Dialysis in intensive care unit patients with acute kidney injury: continuous therapy is superior. Clin J Am Soc Nephrol. 2007;2:597-600.
3. Soni SS, Nagarik AP, Adikey GK, et al. Using continuous renal replacement therapy to manage patients of shock and acute renal failure. J Emerg Trauma Shock. 2009;2(1):19-22.
4. Berbece AN, Richardson RM. Sustained low-efficiency dialysis in the ICU: cost, anticoagulation, and solute removal. Kidney Int. 2006;70:963-8.

5. Brendolan A, Bellomo R, Ronco C. Multiple-organ support therapy for the critically Ill patient. In: Ronco C, Bellomo R, Kellum J (Eds). Critical Care Nephrology, 2nd edition. Saunders Elsevier; 2009. pp. 1571-7.
6. Kaplan AA. Therapeutic plasma exchange: a technical and operational review. J Clin Apher. 2013;28(1): 3-10.
7. Cerda J, Tolwani A, Gibney N, et al. Renal replacement therapy in special settings: extracorporeal support devices in liver failure. Semin Dial. 2011;24(2):197-202.
8. Clark E, Molnar AO, Joannes-Boyau O, et al. High-volume hemofiltration for septic acute kidney injury: a systematic review and meta-analysis. Crit Care. 2014;18(1):R7.
9. Livigni S, Bertolini G, Rossi C, et al. Efficacy of coupled plasma filtration adsorption (CPFA) in patients with septic shock: a multicenter randomised controlled clinical trial. BMJ Open. 2014;4(1):e003536.
10. Payen DM, Guilhot J, Launey Y, et al. Early use of polymyxin B hemoperfusion in patients with septic shock due to peritonitis: a multicenter randomized control trial. Intensive Care Med. 2015;41(6): 975-84.

CHAPTER 5

# Indications and Timing of RRT in AKI

Sunitha Binu Varghese

## INTRODUCTION

Acute kidney injury (AKI) is common, occurring in more than 50% of intensive care unit (ICU) patients, and is associated with a substantial increase in mortality.[1] Renal replacement therapy (RRT) is an important component in the armamentarium of management of severe AKI. Though much research has gone into various aspects of management of these patients, there are many controversial and challenging aspects which have not yet been finalized. One of the foremost is the optimal timing of RRT in patients who do not manifest life-threatening complications of AKI. This still remains a top research priority.

## WHY THE CONTROVERSY?

There are many factors responsible for uncertainties surrounding the identification of the ideal time for RRT initiation:

- Acute kidney injury in critically ill patients is a complex syndrome showing heterogeneity in the presentation primarily because of multifactorial etiology. The goals of RRT will vary according to the etiology and depending on whether it is acute onset or acute on chronic kidney disease.
- Acute kidney injury in critically ill patients usually occurs as part of multiorgan dysfunction syndrome (MODS). The early stages of AKI are usually asymptomatic or have a subtle presentation and hence recognition is already delayed.
- *Definition of "Timing" related to RRT initiation* is without a consensus, leading to heterogeneity in the definitions of "early" and "late" and hence interpreting the available literature on this issue is really challenging.[2]
- Renal replacement therapy is an invasive procedure and is not without the risk of adverse consequences related to vascular access, anticoagulation, and hemodynamics.
- So, though early RRT has potential benefits, it may lead to subjecting some patients, who may spontaneously recover in the course of time, to unnecessary risks of an invasive procedure.[3]
- At the same time, waiting too long to commence RRT may lead to loss of valuable time and lead to poorer prognosis.

- Nonavailability of prediction scores or validated biomarkers at present to predict recovery of AKI or future need of RRT.

The *furosemide stress test (FST)*[4] is emerging as a dynamic tool which may enable to predict which early AKI patients will progress to higher stages of AKI and therefore RRT may be initiated early. FST is performed by intravenously administering furosemide (1 or 1.5 mg/kg) in euvolemic AKI patients followed by measurement of the urine output in the following 2 hours. The ideal cutoff predicting nonprogression and hence probable recovery is a urine volume of >200 mL (100 mL/hr). The feasibility of this test has successfully tested by Lumlertgul et al. Further validation requires large scale studies.

## GOALS OF RRT IN ICU SETTINGS[5] (BOX 1)

The decision pertaining to optimal indications and timing of RRT in ICU requires defining goals of this modality for which currently there is no consensus for various reasons, e.g. much of the RRT utilization is extrapolated from use of dialysis in end-stage renal disease (ESRD) where the goals of RRT are to avoid dialysis as far as possible, whereas in ICU the goal is to prevent or minimize worsening of AKI and/or uremic complications and also to facilitate other medical interventions like nutrition, antibiotics, and blood products.

## CURRENT PRACTICE

Various studies have pointed out that there is wide variation in practice among physicians, across institutions and among nations, because of absence of concrete data with regards to optimal timing of RRT. Clinicians at present consider RRT only when there are life-threatening indications *(classic or absolute indications)* or uremic symptoms or progression in biochemical parameters like blood urea nitrogen (BUN) and serum creatinine *(preemptive indications).*

Nonclinical factors are also noted to play an important role like time of the day that laboratory and clinical results became available, patient's age, comorbidities, and response to diuretic challenge, etc.[6] In daily clinical practice, logistical or organizational aspects of a given institution are also important factors influencing timing.

In an international survey of intensivists across Europe, a new aspect observed was RRT initiation when urinary output is less than 0.5 mL/kg/hr for at least 6 hrs (Risk category of RIFLE (risk, injury failure, loss of kidney function and end stage kidney disease) classification of AKI). This highlights the increasing preference among intensivists for *"Early RRT"* though there is not much evidence favoring this.[7]

**Box 1:** Goals of renal replacement therapy in acute kidney injury (AKI).

- Achieve and maintain fluid and electrolyte balance
- Acid–base and solute homeostasis
- Prevent or minimize worsening of AKI and or uremic complications
- Permit renal recovery
- Facilitate fluid allowances for nutrition, medication, and obligatory fluid intake

## INDICATIONS FOR THE INITIATION OF RRT IN AKI[4,8]

There is no controversy regarding urgent initiation of RRT in patients who present with life-threatening complications of severe AKI (Classic indications). The dilemma is about RRT initiation in patients with severe AKI who do not have these indications.

### Conventional or Absolute or Classic Indications (Box 2)

**Box 2:** Absolute indications (In the absence of contraindications to renal replacement therapy).

- Refractory hyperkalemia
- Refractory acidemia and metabolic acidosis
- Refractory pulmonary edema due to fluid overload
- Symptoms or complications attributable to uremia
- Overdose or toxicity from a dialyzable drug or toxin

- *Refractory hyperkalemia*: Hyperkalemia is frequently seen in patients with AKI. There is no agreement on the threshold at which dialysis should be initiated in AKI. RRT is recommended in patients with severe hyperkalemia, refractory to the usual pharmacological measures. The decision also depends on the acuity of development of hyperkalemia and cardiac effects. Hemodialysis is the preferred modality in these patients.
- *Fluid overload as an indication for RRT*: Positive fluid balance is common in the ICU because of the fluid resuscitation strategies for hemodynamic optimization in patients with hypotension and shock. Observational studies have shown that the severity of volume overload at the time of RRT initiation is associated with increased mortality risk.[4] Removal of fluid and optimization of fluid balance is also associated with improved outcomes.
- Renal replacement therapy is to be initiated if there is evidence of fluid overload which is unresponsive to diuretics especially in patients with low physiological reserve, e.g. congestive heart failure and patients with acute lung injury.
- *Refractory metabolic acidosis*: Metabolic acidosis frequently accompanies AKI in critically ill patients. Usually RRT is not required to manage metabolic acidosis unless there is associated volume overload or hyperkalemia. There is no specific threshold of pH to decide the exact timing of RRT but usually an intractable acidosis (pH below 7.15) is considered as an indication for RRT.
- *Azotemia and or uremic complications*: Progressive azotemia itself is frequently used as an indication to initiate RRT in ICU. There is no specific urea threshold at present but a blood urea of 56–112 mg/dL is often used as a trigger which actually represents the current clinical practice.
- Oliguria/anuria is also often a reason to start early RRT in ICU because it leads to volume overload.
- Uremic complications like bleeding, pericarditis, and encephalopathy are other indications for RRT in AKI similar to ESRD patients.
- *Overdose or toxicity from a dialyzable drug or toxin* is another indication for RRT.

### Relative or Non AKI Indications[9]

- Limited physiologic reserve to tolerate the consequences of AKI like fluid accumulation in patients with underlying congestive cardiac failure.

- Advanced nonrenal organ dysfunction worsened by excessive fluid accumulation like adult respiratory distress syndrome.
- Extracorporeal carbon dioxide removal during permissive hypercapnia.
- Anticipated solute burden (tumor lysis syndrome, rhabdomyolysis, intravascular hemolysis).
- For immunomodulation—RRT in sepsis came as an attractive hypothesis because of its ability to remove inflammatory mediators. There is at present no benefit of resorting to this procedure.[9]

### Relative Contraindications[9]

- Patients who are on palliative care
- The futility of further treatment is known to the treating physician
- Patients who have refused long-term dialysis but at present are having AKI with no probability of recovery.

## RATIONALE FOR EARLY AND LATE RRT (TABLE 1)

In the absence of absolute indications, commencing RRT at an earlier stage of AKI is *theoretically* associated with early achievement of homeostasis with regards to acid-base and electrolytes, removal of uremic toxins, and prevention of fluid accumulation and overload. Earlier RRT can also lead to avoidance or prevention of overt complications of AKI.

*Rationale behind late or conservative approach* to RRT is the possibility that we may be buying time to enable the kidney to recover spontaneously thereby avoiding RRT and associated risks like vascular access and anticoagulation associated complications, intradialytic hypotension, electrolyte imbalance, increased bedside workload, and healthcare costs.

## LITERATURE REVIEW

In the absence of life-threatening complications, the optimal timing for RRT initiation in patients with severe AKI is open to ambiguity. Evidence favoring *"Early RRT"* has come mostly from observational and cohort studies as is clear from the two meta-analyses:

**Table 1:** Benefits and risks of *"Early"* initiation of renal replacement therapy (RRT).

| *Benefits of Early RRT* | *Risks of Early RRT* |
|---|---|
| • Improved *volume control*<br>• Quicker restoration of *acid–base homeostasis*<br>• Earlier control of *electrolyte/metabolic derangement*<br>• Control of complications of *uremia*<br>• Avoidance of unnecessary or excessive diuretic exposure<br>• Accelerated removal of small- and middle-sized molecules<br>• Avoidance of morbidity associated with *"wait for a complication"* approach to initiation of RRT | • Complications associated with the *dialysis catheter*<br>• Risk of iatrogenic episodes of *hemodynamic instability*<br>• Risk of excess clearance/subtherapeutic levels of *vital medications*<br>• Risk of excess loss of *essential substances*<br>• *Electrolyte* imbalance with potential for arrhythmias<br>• *Anticoagulation*-related complications<br>• Unnecessary exposure to RRT in some patients<br>• Increased bedside workload for providers, resource use, and *costs* |

- The first meta-analysis by *Seabra et al.* analyzed 23 studies [only five randomized controlled trials (RCTs)] and reported improved survival with early RRT initiation.[10]
- The second was a meta-analysis of 15 studies (only two RCTs) by *Karvellas et al.* which reported a significant reduction of mortality risk at 28 days with "Early" RRT.[11]

Both the meta-analyses were associated with significant heterogeneity with variable quality and had only few RCTs.

Major RCTs which have compared *"Early" vs. "Delayed"* strategies of RRT initiation have yielded conflicting results.

Evidence from two recent meta-analyses is in favor of *"Late RRT"*:
- First is a meta-analysis of nine high quality studies (Six RCTs, three cohorts) selected after a systematic review of 36 studies, by *Wiestra et al.* which concluded that early RRT initiation in critically ill patients with AKI did not improve survival thereby supporting conservative approach in initiation of RRT.[12]
- Second is an updated meta-analysis of 10 randomized trials by *Bhatt et al.* which showed no significant difference between the two groups on all-cause mortality and dialysis dependence. But there was high heterogeneity in the included trials.[13]

High hopes were pinned on the two largest RCTs till date, AKIKI (Artificial Kidney Initiation in Kidney Injury) by Gaudry et al. and ELAIN (Effect of Early vs. Delayed Initiation of Renal Replacement Therapy on Mortality in Critically Ill Patients With Acute Kidney Injury) study by Zarbock et al. published concurrently but which showed contradictory results.[14,15]

*Conclusions from the AKIKI study*: The study did not demonstrate significant difference with regard to 60-day mortality between the two strategies. Moreover, delayed strategy averted the need for RRT in an appreciable number of patients. Compared with the delayed-strategy group, catheter-related infections and hypophosphatemia were more common in the early-strategy group.

*Conclusions from the ELAIN study*: Early RRT reduced the 90-day mortality rate compared with delayed RRT. The study also demonstrated that early RRT was associated with greater kidney recovery, shorter durations of RRT dependence, mechanical ventilation, and hospitalization.

AKIKI and ELAIN, the results of these two trials were totally discordant. There are many reasons why these two studies have limited comparability. One of the major reasons for this was the basic differences in the design of the two studies.

Though AKIKI and ELAIN trials have failed in reaching a consensus on the issue, they have definitely helped us in understanding the needs of future studies in this regard.

The recently published RCT (IDEAL-ICU study) involving 500 patients of sepsis with severe AKI comparing *"Early" vs. "Delayed"* initiation of RRT showed no survival benefit with the former.[16]

## CURRENT RECOMMENDATIONS

### Kidney Disease Improving Global Outcome (KDIGO) Clinical Practice Guideline for Acute Kidney Injury (2012)[4]

- Initiate RRT emergently when life-threatening changes in fluid, electrolyte, and acid–base balance exist (Not Graded).

- Consider the broader clinical context, the presence of conditions that can be modified with RRT and trends of laboratory tests—rather than single BUN and creatinine thresholds alone—when making the decision to start RRT. (Not Graded)

### National Institute for Health and Care Excellence (NICE)[17]

Refer adults, children, and young people immediately for RRT if any of the following is not responding to medical management:

- Hyperkalemia
- Metabolic acidosis
- Complications of uremia (i.e. pericarditis, encephalopathy)
- Fluid overload
- Pulmonary edema.

## APPROACHES TO OPTIMIZE TIMING OF RRT

In the absence of an accepted consensus, the right time and the right indication to start RRT, in critically ill patients with AKI, has to be decided on individual basis taking into consideration various patient-related factors or variables. So an *Algorithmic Approach* or *Demand-Capacity Framework Model,* as given below, will aid in easy decision making for the intensivists.

### Algorithmic Approach to Initiation of RRT in Critically Ill Patients with AKI[9,18]

*Step I:*

- Look for the presence of life-threatening complications or absolute indications in a patient diagnosed with AKI refractory to medical measures.
- If any one or more complications or absolute indications are present then *Start RRT,* otherwise, *Step II.*

*Step II:*

- Optimize the hemodynamic profile by assessing intravascular volume, cardiac output, mean arterial pressure, intra-abdominal pressure and doing appropriate interventions like treating fluid deficits if any.
- Strategies to prevent further deterioration of kidney function (e.g. discontinue or avoid nephrotoxins).

*Step III: Assessment at regular intervals:*

- Response to resuscitation
- Severity of AKI and baseline kidney function
- Severity of underlying illness
- Trend in laboratory parameters like BUN, serum creatinine
- Development of other organ dysfunction.

*Step IV:*

If persistent or worsening AKI, *Consider Initiating RRT* in the presence of at least one of the following:

- Progressive fluid accumulation
- Complications of fluid overload, e.g. pulmonary edema
- Urine output <0.5 mL/kg/hr for 6–12 hrs or <500 mL/24 hr
- Progressive metabolic acidosis (e.g. pH <7.25)
- Progression or worsening of nonrenal dysfunction
- Anticipated burden of solute burden (e.g. tumor lysis syndrome, rhabdomyolysis)

Go back to *Step III* if there is no worsening or patient starts showing improvement.

(RRT should not be considered at any stage if it is inappropriate or futile or end of life concerns are there)

## RRT Support Based on Demand Capacity Framework[19,20]

This model has been proposed by Mehta RL et al.[19]

*Capacity* refers to the infinite capability of the kidney to support other organ functions. In AKI, the excretory capacity of the kidney is reduced and if unable to meet the demands placed on it, this results in a mismatch.

*Demand* is a dynamic process and refers to the load placed on the kidney function, which predominantly depends on three sets of factors:

1. Severity of the acute illness as assessed by various scoring systems (SOFA, SAPS)
2. Volume and solute load
3. Underlying comorbidities associated with limited physiologic reserve to tolerate the consequences of AKI, e.g. age, congestive cardiac failure, chronic kidney disease, chronic lung disease, and chronic liver disease.

The *Demand-Capacity Balance* has to be evaluated on daily basis and decision for optimal timing of RRT has to be taken depending on the mismatch between demand and capacity.

Based on this concept, there can be two extremes of scenarios:

1. A patient with early stage of AKI may still require "renal support therapy" if the demands exceed the capacity.
2. A patient in late stage of AKI may still follow a conservative approach if there is no mismatch between demand and supply.

Figure 1 illustrates RRT support based on underlying demand and capacity framework.

The 17th Acute Disease Quality Initiative (ADQI) Consensus Conference was conducted at Asiago, Italy, in 2016 on "Patient Selection and Timing of Continuous Renal Replacement Therapy". The highlights were:[20]

- *Consensus statement 1*: Acute RRT should be considered when metabolic and fluid demands exceed total kidney capacity.

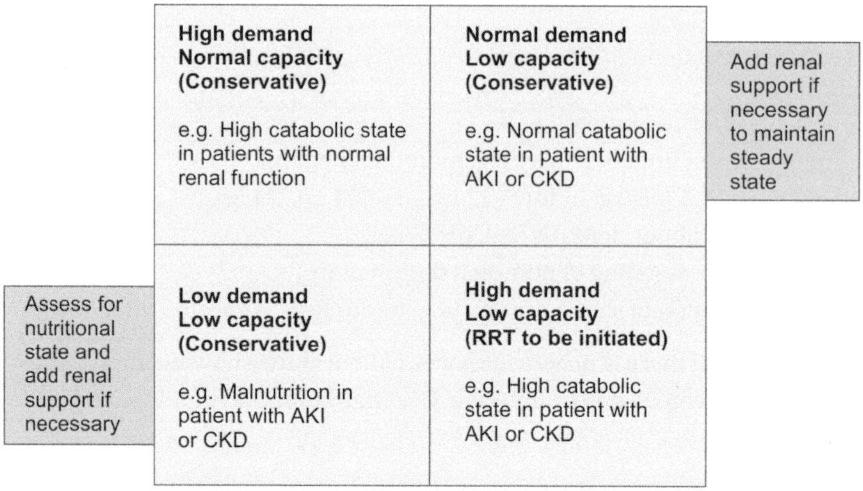


**Fig. 1:** Decision making for RRT based on demand capacity framework.
(AKI: acute kidney injury; CKD: chronic kidney disease; RRT: renal replacement therapy)

- *Consensus statement 2*: Demand for kidney function is determined by nonrenal comorbidities, the severity of the acute disease, and solute and fluid burden.
- *Consensus statement 3*: For patients requiring multiple types of organ support, decisions about initiating or withholding RRT should be considered together with other therapies.
- *Consensus statement 4*: Once the decision to initiate RRT has been made, the therapy should be started as soon as possible, typically within less than 3 hours.

## CONCLUSION

The optimal time to initiate RRT in patients with severe AKI, without the conventional indications, is at present unknown. The decision making process is quite complex in absence of a consensus. The ambiguity will continue till definitive recommendations can be laid down. This is possible only with high-quality RCTs which will strengthen the present evidence and reduce the variability in clinical practice. The available literature at present especially after the IDEAL-ICU study does not seem to favor "*Early*" initiation of RRT in critically ill patients without any urgent or absolute indications.

In the present scenario where there is no consensus and there are no reliable validated parameters to predict the nonrecovery of kidney function and need of RRT in future, decision to start RRT should be individualized taking into account:
- The trends in AKI severity and laboratory parameters
- The severity and reversibility of the underlying illness and associated acute organ dysfunction
- Underlying comorbidities impacted by AKI/fluid overload
- The physiologic reserve and tolerance to fluid overload
- Risk vis-à-vis benefits of RRT

- Resource allocation and costs
- Wishes of patient and family members.

The agenda for research in this context should be adequately powered, RCTs with a clear definition of *"Early"* and integrating novel biomarkers which can predict the recovery or progressive deterioration of kidney function. Till then, the clinically based algorithm or the demand–capacity model discussed above can be used to guide clinicians on when to consider initiation of RRT.

## REFERENCES


1. Hoste EA, Bagshaw SM, Bellomo R, et al. Epidemiology of acute kidney injury in critically ill patients: the multinational AKI-EPI study. Intensive Care Med. 2015;41(8):1411-23.
2. Bagshaw SM, Wald R. (2017). Timing of renal replacement therapy initiation in AKI. [online] Renal and Urology News. Available from http://www.renalandurologynews.com/nkf-2017-spring-meeting/acute-kidney-injury-renal-replacement-therapy-initiation-timing/article/642602 [Last accessed June 2019].
3. Schiffl H. Timing of renal replacement therapy in acute kidney injury: Shedding new light on an old controversy. Indian J Crit Care Med. 2018;22(10):730-2.
4. Schetz M, Forni LG, Joannidis M. Does this patient with AKI need RRT? Intensive Care Med. 2016;42: 1155-8.
5. Kidney disease: Improving Global Outcomes (KDIGO) Acute Kidney Injury Work Group. KDIGO clinical practice guideline for acute kidney injury. Kidney Int Suppl. 2012;2,89-115.
6. Clark E, Wald R, Walsh M, et al. Canadian Acute Kidney Injury (CANAKI) Investigators. Timing of initiation of renal replacement therapy for acute kidney injury: a survey of nephrologists and intensivists in Canada. Nephrol Dial Transplant. 2012;27(7):2761-7.
7. Legrand M, Darmon M, Joannidis M, et al. Management of renal replacement therapy in ICU patients: an international survey. Intensive Care Med. 2013;39:101-8.
8. Joannidis M, Forni LG. Clinical review: Timing of renal replacement therapy. Crit Care. 2011;15(3):223.
9. Bagshaw SM, Wald R. Strategies for the optimal timing to start renal replacement therapy in critically ill patients with acute kidney injury. Kidney Int. 2017;91:1022-32.
10. Seabra VF, Balk EM, Liangos O, et al. Timing of renal replacement therapy initiation in acute renal failure: a meta-analysis. Am J Kidney Dis. 2008;52(2):272-84.
11. Karvellas CJ, Farhat MR, Sajjad I, et al. A comparison of early versus late initiation of renal replacement therapy in critically ill patients with acute kidney injury: a systematic review and meta-analysis. Crit Care. 2011;15(1):R72.
12. Wierstra BT, Kadri S, Alomar S, et al. The impact of "early" versus "late" initiation of renal replacement therapy in critical care patients with acute kidney injury: a systematic review and evidence synthesis. Crit Care. 2016;20(1):122.
13. Bhatt GC, Das RR. Early versus late initiation of renal replacement therapy in patients with acute kidney injury-a systematic review & meta-analysis of randomized controlled trial. BMC Nephrol. 2017;18(1):78.
14. Gaudry S, Hajage D, Schortgen F, et al. AKIKI Study Group. Initiation strategies for renal-replacement therapy in the intensive care unit. N Engl J Med. 2016;375:122-33.
15. Zarbock A, Kellum JA, Schmidt C, et al. Effect of early vs. delayed initiation of renal replacement therapy on mortality in critically ill patients with acute kidney injury: the ELAIN randomized clinical trial. JAMA. 2016;315:2190-9.

16. Saber D Baber, Raphael Clere-Jehl, et al. Timing of Renal-Replacement Therapy in Patients with Acute Kidney Injury and Sepsis. N Engl J Med. 2018;379:1431-42.
17. National Institute for Health and Care Excellence (NICE). (2013). (2013). (Online) Acute kidney injury: prevention, detection and management. Available from https://www.nice.org.uk/guidance/cg169/ [Last accessed June 2019].
18. Bagshaw SM, Cruz DN, Gibney RT, et al. A proposed algorithm for initiation of renal replacement therapy in adult critically ill patients. Crit Care. 2009;13(6):317.
19. Mehta RL. Challenges and pitfalls when implementing renal replacement therapy in the ICU. Crit Care. 2015;19:S9.
20. Ostermann M, Joannidis M, Pani A, et al. Patient Selection and Timing of Continuous Renal Replacement Therapy on behalf of 17th ADQI International Consensus Group. Blood Purif. 2016;42:224-37.

CHAPTER 6

# Vascular Access for Renal Replacement Therapy

*Tarun K Jeloka*

## INTRODUCTION

About 13.5% of intensive care unit (ICU) patients will require some form of renal replacement therapy (RRT).[1] Any form of extracorporeal therapy will require a vascular access to provide rapid blood flow.

Vascular access can be permanent or temporary:

- Permanent access for RRT includes arteriovenous fistula or grafts.
- Temporary access includes central venous catheters—nontunneled catheters and tunneled or cuffed catheters.

In ICUs, central venous catheters are the predominant accesses for extracorporeal therapies.

*Tunneled catheters* are semipermanent and have life more than nontunneled catheters but definitely lesser than permanent accesses. Tunneled catheter requires comparatively bigger procedure, usually requires operating room, and is more expensive than nontunneled catheters.

*Nontunneled catheters* are indicated when need for therapy is short, usually less than a week, or if the patient is too critical to undergo procedure for tunneled catheter. Nontunneled catheter is the one desired when there is emergency or urgent need for dialysis. These nontunneled catheters can be switched to tunneled catheters when need for dialysis is prolonged and patient is relatively stable to undergo the procedure.

In this review, we will focus predominantly on nontunneled dual lumen catheters as they are the most frequently used temporary catheters in ICU and also recommended by Kidney Disease Improving Global Outcomes (KDIGO).[2] This review is a brief overview of vascular access and its complications and not intended for detailed discussion, for which the author recommends other review articles from the "References".

## CATHETERS

There are many different types of catheters available but none have been proven to be significantly superior to others in a well-designed study. Even triple-lumen catheters, when compared with typical double-lumen catheter, have similar blood flow rates and infection

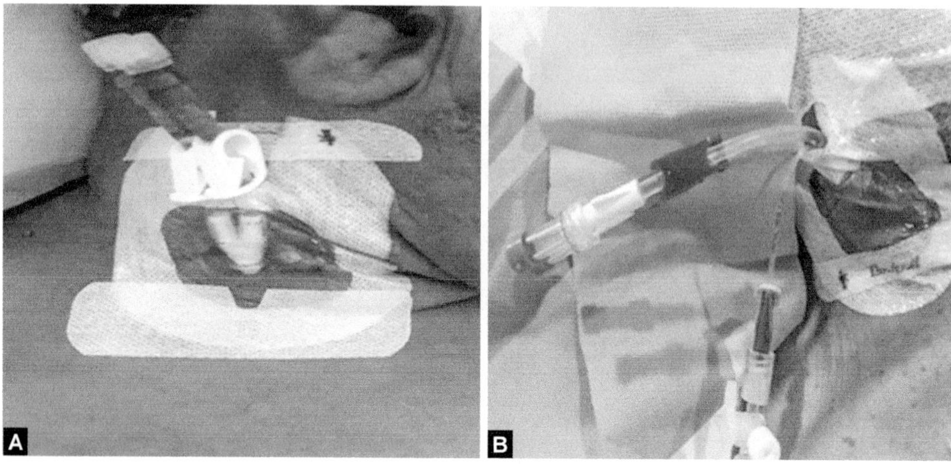

**Figs. 1A and B:** Temporary/nontunneled catheter—double-lumen and triple-lumen catheters. *(For color version, see Plate 3)*

rates (Figs. 1A and B). In the catheter, generally "arterial" opening is proximal or at sides whereas "venous" opening is distal or at the tip.

Kidney Disease Improving Global Outcomes describes various options of catheter sizes and location of insertion.[2] As per Poiseuille's law, blood flow through the catheter is directly proportional to radius and inversely proportional to length of catheter. Hence, there is always a balance between size and location of catheter. Hence, the most preferred site of insertion is right internal jugular, being straight with low turbulence and short distance with low resistance, as compared to any other site. Subclavian veins are best avoided as per guidelines, as it has highest risk of stenosis and insertion related complications.

There are different types of catheters with different lengths, diameter, tips, and lumens.
- Length should be adequate to reach a low pressure area in the central vein.
- Diameter should be adequate to allow a flow of more than 300–400 mL/min.
- Tip of catheter has variations so as to allow minimal *"recirculation"* (Recirculation is mixing of dialyzed blood with venous blood because of inadequate blood flow and is an important reason for ineffective dialysis dose). Split tip catheters (in tunneled catheters) are good but difficult to introduce in ICU. Step tip or shot gun catheters are considered best for ICU patients (Fig. 2). Cycle-C or kidney-shaped lumens are considered optimal as compared to co-axial or double-D (Fig. 2). At times, triple-lumen catheters are also used where the third lumen is used for medications and drawing of blood for tests. However, one should be careful in administering drugs while on dialysis, as the medicine might get dialyzed into the dialyzer lowering its efficacy.

The placement of dialysis access is similar to that of central venous access placement by Seldinger technique. The usual sites are internal jugular, femoral, and subclavian veins. Where available, ultrasound guidance is always suggested while putting any dialysis catheter (especially in internal jugular, where success rate is better and complication rates lower). The tip should be confirmed either by fluoroscopy or chest X-ray film. Malposition is common, 25–40%, which can

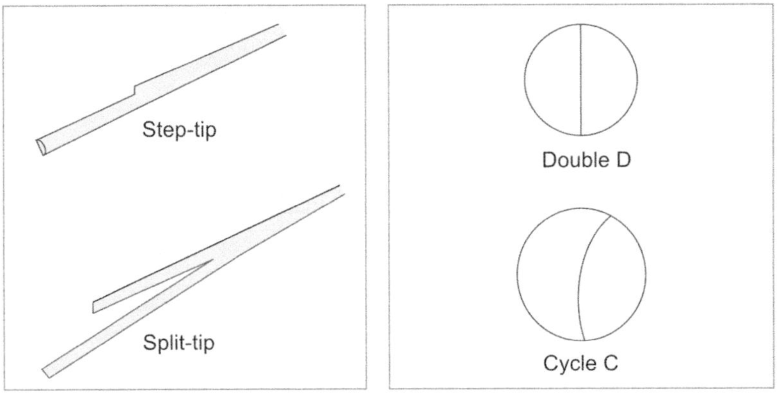


**Fig. 2:** Catheter tip designs.

be managed when fluoroscopy is used. The right internal jugular vein should be the preferred site for dialysis catheter. Left internal jugular has higher rates of infection. Subclavian veins have higher risk of stenosis, insertion-related complications, and are better avoided. Femoral, for short period, is an alternative and rarely, external jugular can also be used.

## Tunneled Catheters

For noncritical patients in ICU, who can be moved to a procedure room, tunneled catheter is preferred as recovery duration from acute kidney injury is difficult to predict. Also, if the recovery is less likely in cases of pre-existing stage 3 or 4 chronic kidney disease, tunneled catheter should be preferred. Tunneled catheters, also called as cuffed catheters, have a cuff which is positioned subcutaneously 1–2 cm from the exit site. This cuff seals off the tunnel and decreases the risk of infection. These catheters are made up of silicone or other flexible polymers like polyurethane, which is less thrombogenic than nontunneled catheters. These catheters may have even larger size like 15.5 to 16 Fr, allowing >400 mL/min of blood flow. There are variety of designs such as coaxial, split-tip etc. for improving the blood flow and reducing the recirculation. However, the long-term functional survival remains the same. Various other modifications like antibiotic-coated catheters have shown to have reduced risk of infection, but heparin-coated catheters have not shown reduction in thrombosis. 1-year catheter survival is 74% and 2-year survival is 43%.[3]

## Nontunneled Catheters

These are made up of polyurethane, polyethylene, polyvinyl chloride or silicone. The outer shaft diameter varies from 8 Fr to 13.5 Fr and provides a flow rate of 300–400 mL/min. Length of catheters can be from 9 cm to as long as 30 cm. Length depends on height of the individual and the point of insertion, with left-sided catheters to have bigger length. The optimal length of catheter for right internal jugular is 12–15 cm, for left internal jugular is 15–20 cm, and for femoral is 19–24 cm.[2] The lifespan of nontunneled catheters is lower than tunneled catheters. Femoral catheters should be removed in less than a week and internal jugular catheters preferably before a month for increasing risk of infection. The incidence of bacteremia 4 weeks following femoral catheter is 29% and that with internal jugular catheter is 10%.[4]

## COMPLICATIONS OF CATHETERS

Complications of dialysis access can be divided into immediate or late complications.

### Immediate Complications

These are generally insertion related. These can be bleeding, hematoma, technique failure, or arterial and venous injury. There can be arterial puncture leading to hematoma, which can be managed with compression. Hematoma can occur in 4.7% of cases. Arterial puncture occurs in 4.2–9.3% of line placements. Arterial injury occurs most commonly with femoral and least with subclavian placements. These complications can be minimized with ultrasound guidance of catheter placement. Catheter malfunction can be early or late. Other rare but serious complications include hemothorax, pneumothorax, air embolism, venous laceration, atrial perforation, inadvertent placement of the catheter into an artery, arteriovenous fistulas, and pseudoaneurysms. Pneumothorax can occur in 1% of catheter insertions and is most common with subclavian. Cardiac complications like arrhythmias and arrest can happen rarely because of guidewire irritating the right atrial myocardium. Many of these rare events will require surgical or vascular intervention, leading to increased morbidity and cost.

#### *Mechanical Malfunction*

It is suspected when there are low flow rates and/or high pressure alarms during dialysis. It is often also diagnosed when blood cannot be withdrawn from the catheter or saline cannot be pushed at the time of initiation. Early catheter malfunction is usually because of mechanical obstruction like kinking of the catheter, tight suture, catheter tip against the vessel wall or thrombosis which may be intra- or extramural. Radiograph imaging including catheterogram may be required to diagnose the cause of malfunction.

Nontunneled catheters are more susceptible to mechanical complications. Many of these early malfunctions may be managed with simple maneuvers. Kink is less likely in temporary catheters and is seen more commonly in tunneled catheters. At times, mild kink can be managed with change in neck position of the patient. Sutures are rarely taken at exit site to manage small vessel bleed from the skin incision. However, it is recommended not to put sutures at the exit site for it can damage the catheter or lead to malfunction if it is too tight. Occasionally, flow is not present at the arterial port, which is on the sides of the catheter tip, because of lying against the vessel wall. Rotation of catheter at times may help. Sometimes, change of ports (interchange of arterial and venous ports) may also help but allows for recirculation and inadequate solute clearance. Early thrombosis may be managed with instillation of heparin or urokinase into the catheter lumen. If the malfunction is still persistent or cause unidentified, it is better to change the catheter as frequent manipulation may result in infection. Late catheter malfunction can happen because of fibrin sheath, thrombosis or central stenosis. Fibrin sheath can occur within 1 week also. It may require fibrinolytics, stripping or catheter removal.

## Late Complications

These can be catheter malfunction, central vein thrombosis and/or stenosis, and catheter infection. Late malfunction (>1 week) can be because of thrombosis or because of fibrin sheath.

### *Central Vein Stenosis/Thrombosis*

In a study, 28% patients developed central vein thrombosis and 14% brachiocephalic vein stenosis within 21 days (range 7–59 days).[4] Stenosis or thrombosis is more frequent with subclavian than internal jugular catheters (15–50% vs. 10–27%).[5-7] These stenosis may remain asymptomatic till arteriovenous fistula is constructed at the same side, when venous return gets affected and it becomes obvious with edema and elevated venous pressure on dialysis. Central vein thrombosis can be managed by anticoagulation, thrombolytic therapy or angioplasty with or without stent.

# CATHETER INFECTION

It includes exit site infection and catheter-related bloodstream infections (CRBSI). This could be a serious complication at times leading to death. The risk of bacteremia with tunneled catheter is 2.3 per 1,000 catheter days.[8] With nontunneled catheters, femoral is associated with highest risk than jugular and then subclavian. Catheter-related infection may need catheter removal and intravenous antibiotic for nontunneled catheters but catheters can be retained in tunneled catheter, unless nonresolving or patient is critical. Measures to minimize dialysis catheter infection include use of antimicrobial agents at exit site, antibiotic lock solution, and eradicating nasal carriage. Antimicrobial coated catheters reduce bacterial colonization. However, it may not last till catheter life, may induce drug-resistant infection, and used more for chronic dialysis.

# MAINTENANCE OF CATHETERS

Maintenance is an important part of catheter care so as to ensure adequate flow and improve lifespan of the catheter. After termination of dialysis, it should be flushed forcefully with 10 mL of saline so as to avoid blood in the lumen which may cause clotting. After flushing, a locking solution should be inserted as per each port volume slowly. Catheter locking solutions are many, like citrate-taurolidine, heparin-gentamicin, heparin alone or citrate alone in different concentrations. This prevents catheter clotting and microbial colonization. However, KDIGO recommends against the use of antibiotic locking solutions for nontunneled catheters in ICU. Daily inspection and transparent dressing with all measures of universal precautions including hand hygiene and barrier precaution will increase the life of functioning catheter. KDIGO recommends against the use of topical antibiotics over the skin insertion site of a nontunneled dialysis catheter in ICU patients because of the risk of superimposed fungal infection and antibiotic resistance.[2]

## Steps in Catheter Care

*Step 1*: While starting dialysis, a trained nurse should be allowed to handle the catheter and another nurse/technician should be managing the dialysis machine.

*Step 2*: The nurse handling the catheter should use mask, cap and sterile gloves, and gloves should be changed if any manipulation is required in between the session.

*Step 3*: Nurse should remove the dressing of the shaft of the catheter and inspect the transparent dressing of the exit site for any evidence of secretions. If any ooze is present, the dressing should be changed. If any erythema or pus at the exit site, it should be informed to the physician and appropriate action taken.

*Step 4*: Both the port caps should be removed and kept soaked in a bowl containing chlorhexidine or at least betadine till the end, when they are re-capped.

*Step 5*: The locking solution should be aspirated from each port one by one by a 10 mL syringe till 1–2 mL blood also comes out, and is discarded. The flow in both the ports is confirmed by aspirating and pushing the blood 2–3 times. Then, both the ports should be flushed with 5–10 mL normal saline forcefully so as to flush the blood from the catheter. The catheter clamp at each port should always remain tight except while aspiration and flushing.

*Step 6*: The dialysis blood tubing is then connected appropriately—arterial port (red ) to arterial line (red) and venous port (blue) to venous line (blue). The clamps are then released so as to allow blood flow for the dialysis.

*Step 7*: At the end of dialysis session, a new pair of sterile gloves should be used and both the ports clamped. Blood tubing is disconnected and handed over to the other nurse/ technician managing thc machine. Both the ports are again flushed with 5–10 mL normal saline forcefully so that blood does not remain in the catheter shaft, which promotes thrombosis and infection.

*Step 8*: Locking solution, either heparin (most commonly used, easily available and cheap) or citrate locking solution, should be instilled in each port as per their volume slowly and clamps tightened. Both the ports are then capped with soaked caps from the bowl.

*Step 9*: The catheter shafts are then wrapped in sterile gauze, to be reused in the same sequence during next dialysis.

## CONCLUSION

Catheters are integral part of dialysis procedure in the ICU department. These are associated with immediate and delayed complications. Due precautions like sterility at insertion, use of ultrasound machine to guide insertion, daily inspection and care, and early removal when not needed are few steps to avoid complications. With limited evidence available in ICU population, it is apt to say that nontunneled catheter with C-shaped lumen of adequate length inserted at right internal jugular with citrate- or taurolidine-based locking solution will provide reasonable life to catheter function.

## REFERENCES

1. Hoste EA, Bagshaw SM, Bellomo R, et al. Epidemiology of acute kidney injury in critically ill patients: the multinational AKI-EPI study. Intensive Care Med. 2015;41(8):1411-23.

2. Kidney Disease: Improving Global Outcomes (KDIGO) Acute Kidney Injury Work Group. KDIGO Clinical practice guideline for acute kidney injury. Kidney Int Suppl. 2012;2:1-138.
3. Mosquera DA, Gibson SP, Goldman MD. Vascular access surgery: a 2-year study and comparison with the Permcath. Nephrol Dial Transplant. 1992;7(11):1111-5.
4. Oliver MJ, Callery SM, Thorpe KE, et al. Risk of bacteremia from temporary hemodialysis catheters by site of insertion and duration of use: a prospective study. Kidney Int. 2000;58(6):2543-5.
5. Oguzkurt L, Tercan F, Torun D, et al. Impact of short-term hemodialysis catheters on the central veins: a catheter venographic study. Eur J Radiol 2004;52(3):293-9.
6. Hernández D, Díaz F, Rufino M, et al. Subclavian vascular access stenosis in dialysis patients: natural history and risk factors. J Am Soc Nephrol. 1998;9(8):1507-10.
7. Schillinger F, Schillinger D, Montagnac R, et al. Post catheterisation vein stenosis in haemodialysis: comparative angiographic study of 50 subclavian and 50 internal jugular accesses. Nephrol Dial Transplant. 1991;6(10):722-4.
8. Saad TF. Bacteremia associated with tunneled, cuffed hemodialysis catheters. Am J Kidney Dis. 1999;34(6):1114-24.

CHAPTER 7

# Choosing Dialyzers and Hemofilters

*Snehal Gaikwad*

## INTRODUCTION

Dialyzer (used synonymously with filter) is the heart of extracorporeal therapies where the molecular exchange of substances between the blood and the dialysis fluid (DF), and ultrafiltration (UF) takes place. The choice of dialyzer in clinical practice is balance between need of the patient, dialyzer performance, and cost, but largely on facilities and local expertise available.

In patients on maintenance hemodialysis (MHD), both small molecular weight solutes and middle molecular and larger sized uremic toxins are accumulated, especially once residual renal function is lost, larger solutes are retained. Hence outcomes of patients on MHD could be improved by increasing middle molecular and larger sized uremic toxin clearance in addition to achieving dialyzer urea adequacy targets. Standard MHD alone is incapable of removing middle molecules adequately, leading to accumulation of such toxins. Hence, newer modalities have evolved including extended/nocturnal hemodialysis and hemodiafiltration in attempt to address this problem. Short-term data with these techniques have shown promising results. Medium cut-off membrane dialyzers which allow diffusive clearance of similar middle molecular weight uremia toxin clearance without increased albumin losses are now available with promising results in current studies; however long-term outcomes need to be studied.

Sepsis is clinical syndrome characterized by a dysregulated immune response to infections that can result in life-threatening organ dysfunction. Renal replacement therapy (RRT) is recommended in septic patients who develop acute kidney injury (AKI) for uremic clearance. Another application for RRT (hemofiltration in particular) in septic AKI patients is the extracorporeal removal of inflammatory mediators. Standard RRT alone is insufficient to decrease serum cytokine levels, which led to the development of more effective extracorporeal techniques, e.g. high volume hemofiltration (HVHF) or very high volume hemofiltration (VHVHF), high cut-off (HCO) membranes, adsorption alone, and coupled plasma filtration adsorption (CPFA) are among the major evolving strategies. Detailed discussion of these modalities is beyond the scope of this chapter, but we will briefly discuss about some special filters used in septic AKI patients, e.g. HCO membrane, Polymyxin B column, and Cytosorb later.

In this chapter, we will briefly discuss about different type of dialyzers, understanding the terminology used when describing dialyzers, and basic considerations when choosing a dialyzer in maintenance dialysis patient and AKI patients.

## Hollow Fiber Dialyzer

Before discussing the components of a hollow fiber dialyzer, let us look at terminology commonly used while describing dialyzer (Table 1).

Large arrays of dialyzers are available for clinical use with several permutations and combinations based on biocompatibility, flux, and surface area of the dialyzer. Essentially a *dialyzer has three components* as shown in Figure 1

The header is the space enclosed by the end cap and the polyurethane potting material that holds the hollow fibers in place and forms a barrier between the blood and dialysate compartments. Blood flows through the fiber lumens and dialysate flows around the external surface of the fibers. Blood and dialysate should flow in opposite directions (counter-current flow) to maximize diffusive solute transfer. The fiber bundle comprises $7–17 \times 10^3$ semipermeable hollow fibers enclosed in an outer housing case. Typical fibers have internal diameter of 200 nm

**Table 1:** Nomenclature of dialyzer components

| | *Terms* | *Definition* |
|---|---|---|
| 1 | Flux | Defined as β2 microglobulin clearance<br>(Earlier permeability was defined as measure of clearance of middle weight molecule, e.g. β2 microglobulin clearance and flux as measure of ultrafiltration capacity)<br>1. Low flux: <10 mL/min<br>2. Mid flux: 10–20 mL/min<br>3. High flux: >20 mL/min |
| 2 | Bio-incompatibility | Sum of specific interactions between blood and the dialyzer membranes or absence of any perturbations in the blood elements |
| 3 | Mass transfer-area coefficient (KoA) | The efficiency of a given dialyzer in removing any solute can be described by a constant referred to as KoA. Denotes the permeability of the mass transfer barrier between blood and dialysate pathways through diffusion. KoA, measured in milliliters per minute, is defined as the maximum possible clearance of a given dialyzer at infinitely large blood and dialysate flow rates.<br>Described in terms of urea clearance<br>1. Low efficiency: KoA <500 mL/min<br>2. Medium efficiency: KoA 500–700 mL/min<br>3. High efficiency: KoA >700 mL/min |
| 4 | Hydraulic permeability (Kuf) | Intrinsic characteristic of dialyzer that regulates the rate and amount of fluid flow across the dialyzer membrane indicated by its ultrafiltration coefficient, (Kuf). Varies considerably and is a function of membrane thickness and pore size. The ultrafiltration coefficient (Kuf) is the volume of plasma water filtered in milliliters per hour for each mm Hg of transmembrane pressure (TMP) |
| 5 | Transmembrane pressure | The rate of ultrafiltration depends on the total pressure difference across the membrane: calculated as the pressure in the blood compartment minus the pressure in the dialysate compartment |

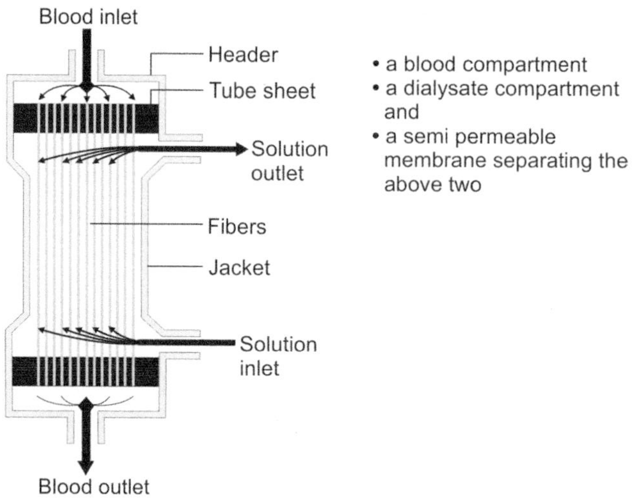


**Fig. 1:** Components of dialyzer.

and wall thickness of 30–40 nm. Fibers may incorporate features, such as undulations, to distribute dialysate flow evenly through the bundle.

*Dialyzer membrane*: It is a semipermeable membrane that allows some solutes to penetrate, while rejecting others by sieving. Dialyzer membrane can be classified based on their chemical composition, efficiency of small-solute (based on urea, 60 Da) removal, efficiency of large-solute (based on β 2-microglobulin, 12 kDa) removal, water or hydraulic permeability (FDA classification), and biocompatibility as mentioned in Table 2 .

## DIALYZER SPECIFICATION SHEET

This sheet provides information about ultrafiltration coefficient (Kuf); clearance of solutes such as urea, creatinine, vitamin $B_{12}$, and phosphate (and occasionally β2-microglobulin); membrane surface area; priming volume; fiber length; and fiber wall thickness. Let us look at a sample dialyzer specification sheet (Table 3).

## SPECIAL FILTERS

In addition to above, there are various other filters used in continuous renal replacement therapy (CRRT), plasma exchange, and other special circumstances, e.g. CRRT filters, plasma filters, HCO membrane filters, and sepsis filters, etc. Discussion of above filters in length is beyond the scope of this chapter. We will discuss each briefly.

### Continuous Renal Replacement Therapy Filters

Continuous renal replacement therapy requires special hemofilter sets. These are part of a complete set, each of which is compatible with specific machines only. Table 4 gives

**Table 2:** Types of dialysis membrane

| *Membrane* | *Membrane name* | *High or Low flux* | *Biocompatibility* |
|---|---|---|---|
| Cellulose | Cuprophane | Low | Low |
| *Semisynthetic cellulose* | | | |
| Cellulose diacetate | Cellulose acetate | Low or high | Intermediate |
| Cellulose triacetate | Cellulose triacetate | High | Good |
| Diethylaminoethyl-substituted cellulose | Hemophane | High | Intermediate |
| *Synthetic polymers* | | | |
| Polymethylmethacrylate | PMMA | High | Good |
| Polyacrylonitrile methacrylate copolymer | PAN | High | Good |
| Polyacrylonitrile methallyl sulfonate copolymer | PAN/AN69 | High | Good |
| Polyamide | Polyflux | High and low | Good |
| Polycarbonate/polyether | Gambrane | High | Good |
| Polyethylene/vinyl alcohol | EVAL | High | Good |
| Polysulfone | Polysulfone | High and low | Good |

*Source:* Floege J, Johnson R, Feehally J (Eds). Comprehensive Clinical Nephrology, 4th edition. US: Saunders, Elsevier Inc; 2010.

**Table 3:** Dialyzer specification sheet for select dialyzers

| *Dialyzer specification* | *FX 8 Low Flux dialyzer* | *FX 80 High Flux Dialyzer* | *FX 800 Hemodiafilters* |
|---|---|---|---|
| UF coefficient (mL/h × mm Hg) | 12 | 59 | 63 |
| Clearance at Qb = 300 mL/min | | | |
| Urea | 254 | 276 | 289 |
| Creatinine | 225 | 250 | 271 |
| Phosphate | 194 | 239 | 262 |
| Vitamin $B_{12}$ | 120 | 175 | 209 |
| Effective surface area ($m^2$) | 1.4 | 1.8 | 1.8 |
| Blood filling volume | 74 mL | 95 mL | 118 mL |
| Membrane material | Helixone | Helixone | Helixone |
| Housing material | Polypropylene | Polypropylene | Polypropylene |
| Potting compound | Polyurethane | Polyurethane | Polyurethane |
| Sterilization method | INLINE Steam | INLINE Steam | INLINE Steam |
| Application | HD | HD/HF/HDF | HD/HDF |

(UF: ultrafiltration, Qb: blood flow, HD: hemodialysis, HF: hemofiltration, HDF: hemodiafiltration)

specifications of hemofilters in common use. The length of the fiber used to prepare CRRT filter is smaller in order to avoid clotting at lower blood flows and high ultrafiltration fraction, inherent to CRRT.

**Table 4:** Specifications of hemofilters in common use for continuous renal replacement therapy (CRRT)[5]

| *Specifications* | *M100* | *M60* | *HF20* | *Ultraflux AV Paed* |
|---|---|---|---|---|
| Membrane | AN69 | Polyarylether sulfone | Polyarylether sulfone | Polysulfone |
| Housing and headers | Polycarbonate | Polycarbonate | Polycarbonate | Polycarbonate |
| Surface area ($m^2$) | 1.0 | 0.6 | 0.2 | 0.2 |
| Appropriate patient weight (kg) | >30 | 11–29 | <8 | <10 kg |
| Blood flow (mL/min) minimum to maximum | 75 and above | 50 and above | 20–100 | No data |
| Set blood volume (mL) | 152 | 93 | 60 | 54 |
| Priming volume (mL) | 66 | 42 | 24 | 18 |
| Maximum TMP mm Hg | 450 | 450 | 500 | 500 |
| Clearance in CVVHD mode with UF = 0 | @Qb = 150 mL/min and effluent 2.5 L/hr | @Qb = 100 mL/min and effluent 1L/hr | @Qb = 50 mL/min and effluent 0.5 L/hr | No data |
| Urea (mL/min) | 41 | 17 | 8.3 | No data |
| Inulin (mL/min) | 23 | 12 | 6.9 | No data |

(CVVHD: continuous venovenous hemodialysis; TMP: transmembrane pressure)

**Table 5:** Specifications of plasma filters in common use

| *Plasma filter specifications* | *PlasmaFlux PSu 1S* | *PlasmaFlux PSu 2S* |
|---|---|---|
| Membrane material | Fresenius Plasmasulfone | Fresenius Plasmasulfone |
| Inner lumen/wall thickness (μm) | 340/70 | 340/70 |
| Effective surface area ($m^2$) | 0.3 | 0.6 |
| Sieving coefficient for molecules up to $2 \times 10^6$ Da | ≈1 | ≈1 |
| Maximum transmembrane pressure (mm Hg) | 100 | 100 |
| Blood filling volume | 36 | 70 |
| Recommended blood flow range (mL/min) | 40–150 | 80–250 |
| Maximum filtrate flow | 20% of effective Qb | 20% of effective Qb |
| Sterilization method | INLINE Steam | INLINE Steam |

## Plasma Filter (Table 5)

A hollow-fiber plasma separator membrane allows only plasma to pass and hold back the formed elements of the blood. The membrane has a sieving coefficient (ratio of concentration in filtrate to blood) between 0.8 and 0.9 for albumin, IgG, IgA, IgM, C3, C4, fibrinogen, cholesterol, and triglycerides [at a blood flow rate of 100 mL per minute and a transmembrane pressure (TMP) of 40 mm Hg].

## Sepsis Filters

### *HCO Membranes*

These membranes have been developed to increase the clearance of inflammatory mediators. The pore sizes of HCO membranes are 2- or 3-fold larger than conventional high-flux membranes (pore size of 0.003–0.006 μm) and one-twentieth of plasma-filtering membranes (pore size of 0.2 μm). These can be used with both diffusive and convective modalities.[1] Major limitation is excessive albumin loss, more when used in convective modalities. HCO membranes have shown to restore immune cell function, attenuate hemodynamic instability, decrease plasma IL-6 levels, and also eliminate larger late-phase inflammatory mediators such as HMGB-1 leading to improvement in ICU patient severity of illness scores as reported by Morgera et al.[2] The High Cut-Off Sepsis study (HICOSS)[3] comparing conventional and HCO membranes was stopped prematurely after enrolment of 81 patients due to a lack of 28-day mortality benefit [HCO (31%) vs. conventional (33%)] and lack of a difference in vasopressor requirement or ICU-LOS.[1] High cut-off hemodialysis is also used in the management of AKI in patients with rhabdomyolysis and multiple myeloma.

Based on the current literature, there is no evidence to support the routine use of HCO hemofiltration in sepsis.

### ***Polymyxin B-immobilized Fiber Column***

Polymyxin B is an antibiotic with strong bactericidal activity against Gram-negative bacteria; it binds to and inactivates endotoxins. Systemic polymyxin B use in humans is restricted because of its nephrotoxicity and neurotoxicity potential. Toraymyxin comprises a plastic column polymyxin B covalently immobilized on the surface of polystyrene derived polypropylene-reinforced conjugated carrier fibers to enable the selective adsorption of circulating endotoxins in the blood.[4]

The evidence supporting use of the polymyxin B-immobilized fiber column (PMX; Toraymyxin) remains mixed. The EUPHRATES trial[5] conducted in North America suggested that less than a 5% mortality difference was recognized in the "per protocol population" (N = 244, 31.9 vs. 36.9%) and that the decrease was not statistically significant.

Table 6 summarizes main studies utilizing polymyxin B immobilized fiber column in Sepsis.[1]

### *CytoSorb*

CytoSorb therapy is based on an extracorporeal blood purification that effectively reduces excessive level of inflammatory mediators. Cartridge contains polystyrene divinylbenzene copolymer beads with a biocompatible polyvinylpyrrolidone coating. Each bead is 300–800 μm in size and each gram of material has a surface area of 850 $m^2$; effective surface area is 40,000 $m^2$. Filter adsorbs molecules < 55 kDa and has low flow resistance.

They can be used in stand-alone mode (hemoperfusion) or inserted within a CRRT circuit (associated with a conventional hemofilter), a cardiopulmonary bypass (CPB) or an extracorporeal membrane oxygenation circuit. CytoSorb removes a wide range of molecules from the blood—pro- and anti-inflammatory cytokines, bilirubin, myoglobin, exotoxins, and also drugs. CytoSorb® (CytoSorbents Corporation, NJ, USA) has been licensed for extracorporeal cytokine removal within the European Union (EU).[14] However, currently there are no recommendations for use in favor of or against such techniques.

Table 7 summarizes studies utilizing CytoSorb cartridge in sepsis patients.[2]

*Modified AN69 (oXiris):* It is a membrane with polyacrylonitrile (polymer of AN69) positively charged with polyethyleneimine.[1]

**Table 6:** Studies on polymyxin B filters

| | *European Pilot study*[6] | *EUPHAS*[7] | *Japan registry*[8] | *ABDO-MIX*[9] | *Japan Registry*[10] | *EUPHARATES*[5] |
|---|---|---|---|---|---|---|
| Year | 2005 | 2009 | 2014 | 2015 | 2016 | 2017 |
| Study design | MCT, pilot, open label, RCT | MCT, open label, prospective RCT | Propensity matched analysis | MCT prospective RCT | Propensity matched analysis | MCT prospective RCT |
| Study population | Surgical patients with intra-abdominal sepsis | Severe sepsis or septic shock due to intra-abdominal infection requiring emergency surgery | Intra-abdominal sepsis patients vs. propensity score-matched pairs | Septic shock due to intra-abdominal infection | AKI due to septic shock patients requiring CRRT | Septic shock with EAA>0.6, MODS>9 |
| Number of cases | 36 (PMX17, control 19) | 64 (PMX 34, control 30) | 1,232 (PMX 642, control 590) | 232 (PMX 119, control 113) | - | 449 (PMX 223, control 226) |
| PMX session Prescribed dose | 1 session × 2 hrs | 2 sessions × 2 hrs each, 24 hrs apart | 1–2 sessions | 2 sessions × 2 hrs each, 24 hrs apart | 1–2 sessions | 2 sessions × 2 hrs each |
| Initiation of PMX treatment | Within 24–48 hrs of diagnosis | Within 24 hrs from surgery | Within 24 hrs from surgery | Within 12 hrs from surgery | Within 24 hrs from CRRT | Within 24 hrs of enrollment |
| Primary endpoint | Improvement in SOFA score | Baseline to 72 hr change in MAP and vasopressor requirement | | 28-day mortality | | 28-day mortality |

*Contd...*

*Contd...*

| | *European Pilot study* | *EUPHAS* | *Japan registry* | *ABDO-MIX* | *Japan Registry* | *EUPHARATES* |
|---|---|---|---|---|---|---|
| Secondary endpoint | Plasma endotoxin and IL-6 levels, 28-day mortality, length of ICU stay, hemodynamic data, need for RRT | $PaO_2/FiO_2$ ratio, change in organ dysfunction (delta SOFA score), 28-day mortality, length of ICU stay and hospital stay, hemodynamic data, need for RRT, all-cause mortality | | 7-,14-,21-, and 90-day mortality, SOFA score variation within first 3 days, time to withdraw inotropes, AEs | | Survival time from baseline to death within 28-day mortality; changes in organ dysfunction, MAP, CVI, renal function from baseline o day 3 |
| Survival/Mortality | PMX 29 % vs. conventional 28%, p = 0. 749 | 28-day mortality significantly reduced in PMX group adjusted HR 0.36, 95% CI p = 0.01<br>Hospital mortality rate significantly reduced in PMX group adjusted HR 0.43, 95% CI p = 0.0026 | 28-day mortality PMX group 17.1% vs. 16.3% in control group, p = 0.696 | 28-day mortality PMX 27.7% vs. conventional 19.5%, p = 0.14 | 28-day mortality<br>PMX group 40.2% vs. 46.8% in control group, p = 0.003<br>28-day mortality<br>PMX group receiving 2 sessions was 35.7 % vs. 42.6% in group treated with one session | 28-day mortality<br>PMX 37.7% vs. Control 34.5 %, p = 0.49 |
| Length of ICU stay | PMX group 13.2 ± 9.4 days vs. control group 17.0 ± 9.4 days | No significant difference | - | No significant difference | - | |
| Hemodynamics | Significant improvement in VP requirement in PMX group | Significant improvement in VP requirement in PMX group | - | No significant difference | No significant difference | No significant difference |

(MAP: mean arterial pressure; AE: adverse event;AKI: Acute kidney injury; CVI: cardiovascular index; CRRT: continuous renal replacement therapy; EAA: endotoxin activity assay; IL-6: interleukin 6; MCT: multicenter trial; MODS: multiple organ dysfunction syndrome; PMX: polymyxin; RCT: randomized control trial; RRT: renal replacement therapy; SOFA sequential organ dysfunction assessment; VP: vasopressor)

**Table 7:** Studies utilizing CytoSorb cartridge in sepsis patients[2]

| | *Friesecke et al. 2017*[12] | *Schädler et al. 2017*[11] | *Kogelmann et al. 2017*[13] |
|---|---|---|---|
| Study design | Prospective intervention, single center | MCT, open label, RCT | Case series |
| Study population | 20 septic shock patients | 97 septic shock patients with ALI or ARDS | 26 septic shock patients with need for RRT |
| Prescribed dose | One session in the pre-filter mode. Further treatments at the discretion of the study physicians | HP vs. no HP (6 h/day for up to 7 days); RRT as clinically indicated in both groups | HP in the pre-filter mode (1–5 treatments) |
| Timing | Within 24 h | | <24 to >48 h (outcomes better in the early group) |
| Primary outcome | VP requirement after 6 hr and 12 hr of CytoSorb therapy | change in normalized IL-6-serum concentrations during study day 1 and 7 | Vasopressor requirement |
| Secondary outcome | SOFA score, resolution of shock and lactate clearance | Multiple organ dysfunction score, ventilation time, time course of oxygenation | Hospital mortality and blood lactate levels |
| Survival | 28-day survival was 45% | 60-day mortality of 44.7% in the treatment group vs. 26.0% in the controls (p = 0.039) | The actual 28-day, ICU, and hospital mortality was 61.54%, 73.08%, and 0.77%, respectively, compared with 89.9% as predicted by APACHE II score |
| Hemodynamics | Significant reduction in VP requirements compared to baseline | – | Significant reduction in VP requirements compared to baseline |
| Other results | Significant reduction in IL-6 and blood lactate levels | No significant reduction in IL-6 | |

(AE: adverse event; ALI: acute lung injury; APACHE II: Acute Physiology and Chronic Health Evaluation II; ARDS: acute respiratory distress syndrome; HP: hemoperfusion; IL: interleukin; ICU: intensive care unit; MCT: multicenter trial; RCT: randomized controlled trial; RRT: renal replacement therapy; ST: standard therapy; VP: vasopressor)

The evidence supporting the use of modified AN69 is limited to case series. In the study reported by Shum et al.,[15] six patients with septic AKI underwent oXiris®-continuous venovenous hemofiltration (CVVH). The results were compared to 24 severity-matched historical controls undergoing standard therapy. The results demonstrated that the SOFA score was reduced after 48 hours CVVH from the value at ICU admission by 38% in the oXiris® group, while it was increased by 3% in the control group. No significant difference was observed in ICU and in-hospital mortality between the two groups.[1,13]

## FACTORS TO CONSIDER WHEN CHOOSING A DIALYZER

The major factors determining which dialyzer to use depends upon the clinical situation of the patient, availability of resources including technical expertise and cost. Basic considerations take into account the flux, efficiency, and biocompatibility of dialyzer.

## Dialyzing Patients with Acute Kidney Injury

Factors to consider in choosing a dialyzer for a patient with AKI patient include membrane composition, dialyzer surface area, and membrane flux.[16]

- *Membrane composition and biocompatibility*: Synthetic dialyzers should be preferred because of their lower immunogenicity and better solute removal. Unmodified cellulosic membranes are associated with greater activation of complement and inflammatory cells.[6] Meta-analyses showed that both patient survival and renal recovery were reduced with unmodified cellulosic dialyzers, but there were no such effects with either modified cellulosic or synthetic membrane dialyzers.[17] Angiotensin converting enzyme (ACE) inhibitors should be avoided in patients when AN69 membrane is used for HD—negatively charged surface of the PAN membrane can activate bradykinins and cause dialyzer reactions.
- *Flux*: Standard HD and sustained low-efficiency dialysis (SLED) can be done using low flux dialyzers. SLED-F and CRRT should use high flux dialyzers and special hemofilter sets. High flux dialyzer with bigger pore size does guarantee better solute/fluid clearance but should only be used with ultrapure water as otherwise there is always a chance of backfiltration of endotoxins/bacteria into the bloodstream.
- *Size of the dialyzer*: The surface area should be as large as possible to optimize clearances. However for the first HD session dialyzer surface area should not exceed 75% of body surface area to avoid disequilibrium syndrome. When treating poisoning or drug toxicity, then a larger sized dialyzer is preferred to increase clearance.
- *Special filters*: There are no recommendations at present regarding use of extracorporeal techniques aiming at elimination of inflammatory mediators involved in pathogenesis of sepsis. Therapy should be tailored to individual patient clinical status.

## Dialyzing End Stage Renal Disease Patients[16]

- *Membrane composition and biocompatibility*: Same as in AKI patients. Biocompatible synthetic or modified cellulosic membranes should be preferred over unmodified cellulose membranes (e.g. Cuprophane). Cuprophane membranes should be used only when other more biocompatible membranes are not available or patient is intolerant to all others.
- *Flux*: Either low flux or high flux membrane can be used for standard HD. High flux dialyzers may be preferred over low flux dialyzers to provide HD under specific situations such as—(1) incident patients, who have lower serum albumin concentrations (<40 g/L) or have diabetes mellitus, and (2) prevalent patients, who have been on HD for more than 4 years or have dialysis related amyloidosis. High flux dialyzer should be used only in facilities where a very high quality of dialysate is ensured at all times.
- *Size of the dialyzer*: Surface area of the dialyzers should be chosen based on the required dialysis dose and the body size of the patient. Large surface area dialyzers should be avoided in pediatric patients and adult patients with small body size especially when initiating MHD. For the first HD session, dialyzer surface area should not exceed 75% of body surface area to avoid disequilibrium syndrome.
- *Dialyzer sterilization method*: The preferred method of sterilization is steam sterilization. Steam-sterilized membranes have been found to improve endothelial cell viability when

compared to ethylene oxide (ETO) or gamma rays-sterilized ones. Hence, use of dialyzers sterilized with ETO should be avoided, steam or gamma sterilized dialyzers are acceptable.

## REFERENCES


1. Ankawi G, Neri M, Zhang J, et al. Extracorporeal techniques for the treatment of critically ill patients with sepsis beyond conventional blood purification therapy: the promises and the pitfalls. Crit Care. 2018;22(1):262.
2. Morgera S, Slowinski T, Melzer C, et al. Renal replacement therapy with high-cutoff hemofilters: impact of convection and diffusion on cytokine clearances and protein status. Am J Kidney Dis. 2004;43(3):444-53.
3. Honore PM, Clark W. Novel therapeutical concepts for extracorporeal treatment of hyperinflammation and sepsis: immunomodulation. approach with a novel high Cut-OFF membrane: the SepteX membrane. In Proceedings of 10th Congress of World Federation of CCU (WFSICCM) 2009. Florence.
4. Shimizu T, Miyake T, Tani M. History and current status of polymyxin B-immobilized fiber column for treatment of severe sepsis and septic shock. Ann Gastroenterol Surg. 2017;1(2):105-13.
5. Dellinger P, Bagshaw SM, Antonelli M, et al. Effect of targeted polymyxin B hemoperfusion on 28-Day mortality in patients with septic shock and elevated endotoxin level the EUPHRATES Randomized Clinical Trial. JAMA. 2018;320(14):1455-1463.
6. Vincent JL, Laterre PF, Cohen J, et al. A pilot controlled study of a polymixin b-immobilized hemoperfusion cartidge in patients with severe sepsis secondary to intra-abdominal infection. Shock. 2005;23(5):400-5.
7. Cruz DN, Antonelli M, Fumagalli R, et al. Early use of polymyxin B hemoperfusion in abdominal septic shock: the EUPHAS randomized controlled trial. JAMA. 2009;301(23):2445.
8. Iwagami M, Yasunaga H, Doi K, et al. Postoperative polymyxin B hemoperfusion and mortality in patients with abdominal septic shock: a propensity-matched analysis. Crit Care Med. 2014;42:1187-93.
9. Payen DM, Guilhot J, Launey Y, et al. Early use of polymyxin B hemoperfusion in patients with septic shock due to peritonitis: a multicenter randomized control trial. Intensive Care Med. 2015;41:975-84.
10. Iwagami M, Yasunaga H, Noiri E, et al. Potential survival benefit of polymyxin B hemoperfusion in septic shock patients on continuous renal replacement therapy: a propensity-matched analysis. Blood Purif. 2016;42(1):9-17.
11. Schädler D, Pausch C, Heise D, et al. The effect of a novel extracorporeal cytokine hemoadsorption device on IL-6 elimination in septic patients: a randomized controlled trial. PLoS One. 2017;12(10):e018701.
12. Friesecke S, Stecher SS, Gross S, et al. Extracorporeal cytokine elimination as rescue therapy in refractory septic shock: a prospective single-center study. J Artif Organs. 2017;20(3):252-9.
13. Kogelmann K, Jarczak D, Scheller M, Drüner M. Hemoadsorption by CytoSorb in septic patients: a case series. Crit Care. 2017;21(1):1-10.
14. Poli EC, Rimmele T, Schneider AG. Hemoadsorption with CytoSorbR. Intensive Care Med. 2019;45(2):236-9.
15. Shum HP, Chan KC, Kwan MC, Yan WW. Application of endotoxin and cytokine adsorption haemofilter in septic acute kidney injury due to Gram-negative bacterial infection. Hong Kong Med J. 2013;19(6):491-7.
16. Rajapurkar MM, Annigeri RA, Gupta A, et al. For ISN guidelines for hemodialysis units work group. Indian Society of Nephrology Guidelines for hemodialysis units. Ind J Nephrol. 2012;22:s13-s15.
17. Haroon S, Davenport A. Choosing a dialyzer: What clinicians need to know. Hemodial Int. 2018;22(S2):S65-S74.

CHAPTER 8

# Set Up and Prescription for CRRT

Ranajit Chatterjee, Ashutosh Garg, Juliet Merlene

## INTRODUCTION

Continuous renal replacement therapy (CRRT) is fast becoming an integral part in the management of critically ill patients in intensive care. It stands apart from its intermittent counterparts like intermittent hemodialysis (IHD) and sustained low efficiency daily dialysis in many aspects including the prescription and dosage. The prescription of CRRT requires an understanding of the different processes of solute removal (which can be applied through various modalities), the circuit, and filter and their properties in order to deliver effective treatment. It also demands knowledge about filter parameters like transmembrane pressure (TMP) and filtration fraction which in turn would determine the filter performance and filter life.

## CRRT MODALITIES (BASED ON PRINCIPLES)

### Slow Continuous Ultrafiltration (Fig. 1)

*The primary therapeutic goal with this modality is safe* management of fluid removal.

*Primary indications*: Fluid overload without significant electrolyte imbalance.

*Principle*: Ultrafiltration

*Therapy characteristics:* No dialysate or substitution solutions, fluid removal only.

*Slow continuous ultrafiltration (SCUF)* is a very useful modality in patients of *diuretic resistant and hemodynamically unstable pulmonary edema.* It is also helpful in removing fluid in cases of *cerebral edema* especially in patient of *acute liver failure and subsequent hepatic encephalopathy.* For solute removal, in encephalopathy, continuous venovenous hemodiafiltration (CVVHDF) or continuous venovenous hemofiltration (CVVH) is preferred.

### Continuous Venovenous Hemofiltration (Fig. 2)

Solute removal and safe management of fluid volume is the primary therapeutic goal.

*Primary indications*: Uremia, severe acid/base or electrolyte imbalance, when removal of larger molecular weight substances is required

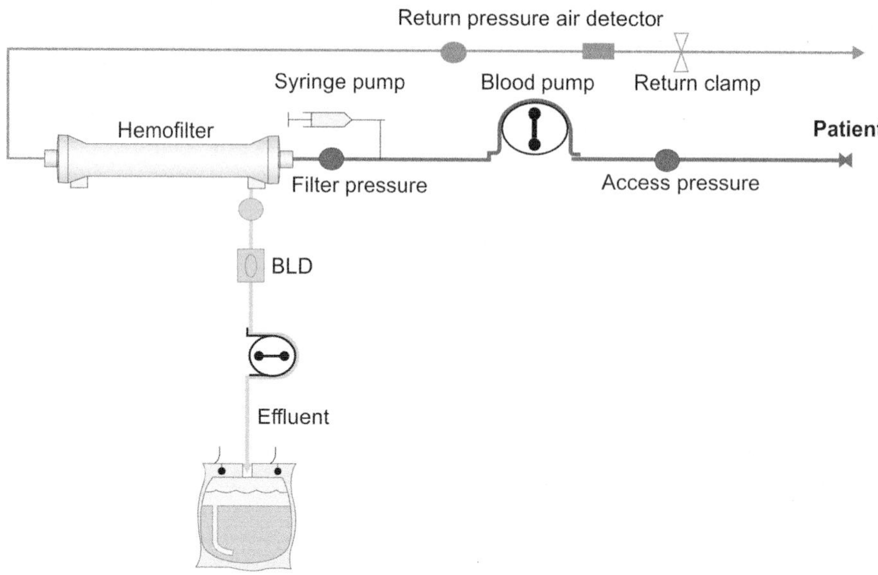


**Fig. 1:** Slow continuous ultrafiltration[6,7]
*(For color version, see Plate 4)*

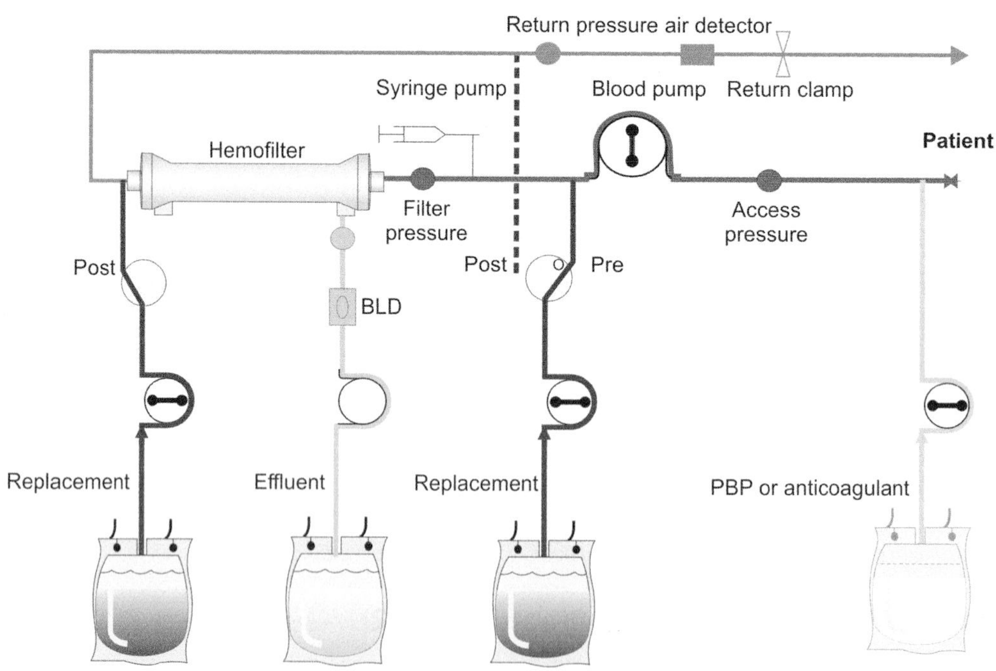


**Fig. 2:** Continuous venovenous hemofiltration[6,7]
*(For color version, see Plate 4)*

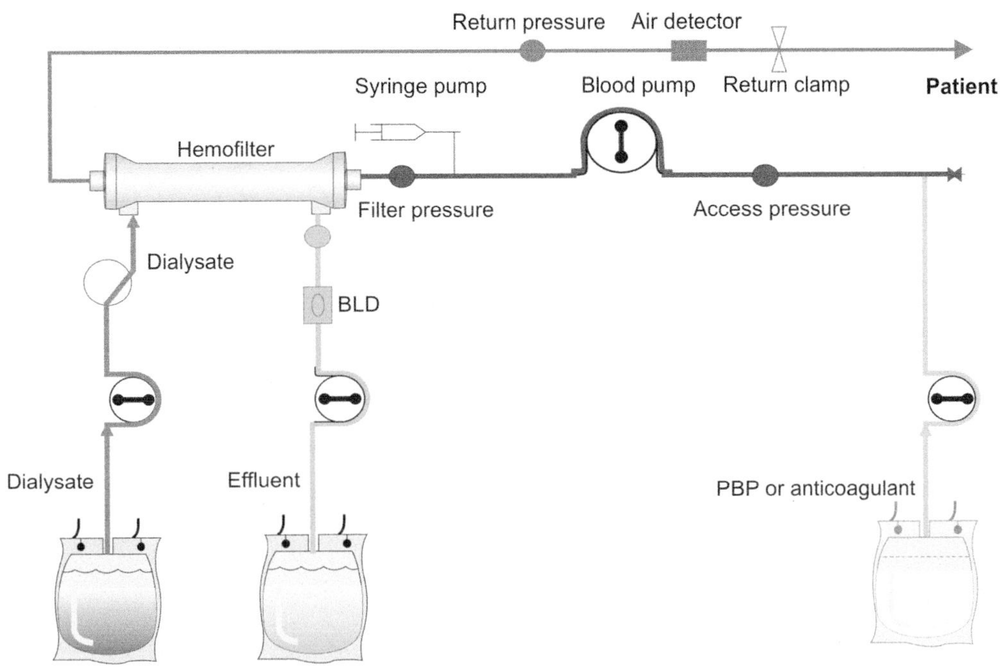


**Fig. 3:** Continuous venovenous hemodialysis[6,7]
*(For color version, see Plate 5)*

*Principle used*: Convection

*Therapy characteristics*: Requires replacement solution to drive convection. No dialysate solution Effective at removing small and middle molecules.

## Continuous Venovenous Hemodialysis (Fig. 3)

*Primary therapeutic goal*: Solute removal and safe management of fluid volume

*Primary indications*: Uremia, severe acid/base or electrolyte imbalance

*Principle used*: Diffusion

*Therapy characteristics*: Requires dialysate solution to drive diffusion. No replacement solution Effective at removing small molecules.

## Continuous Venovenous Hemodiafiltration (Fig. 4)

*Primary therapeutic goal*: Solute removal and safe management of fluid volume

*Primary indications*: Uremia, severe acid/base or electrolyte imbalance, when removal of large molecular weight substances is required

*Principle used*: Diffusion and convection

*Therapy characteristics*: Requires dialysate fluid and replacement solution to drive diffusion and convection

Effective at removing small, medium, and large molecules

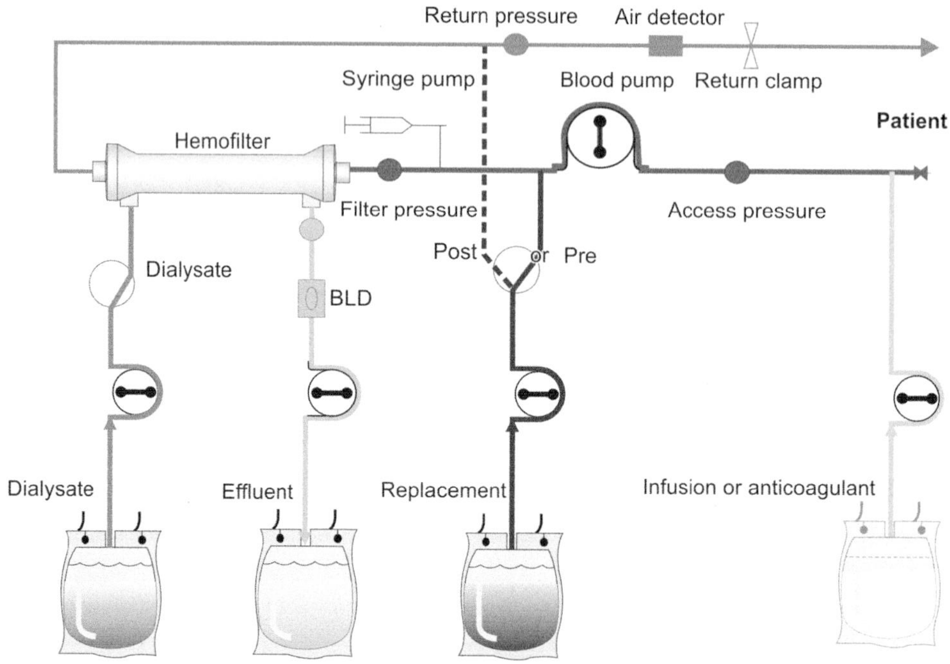


**Fig. 4:** Continuous venovenous hemodiafiltration [6,7]
*(For color version, see Plate 5)*

## COMPONENTS FOR SET UP OF CRRT (FIG. 5)

For setting up of CRRT, the following components would be needed as prerequisites.

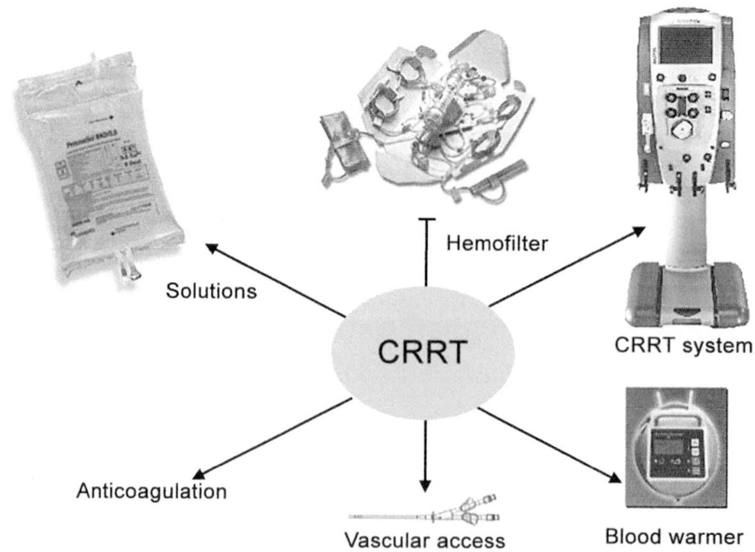


**Fig. 5:** Components of CRRT[8]
*(For color version, see Plate 6)*

## Vascular Access

Vascular access is a basic prerequisite to perform any type of extracorporeal therapy. Access is particularly important in CRRT where catheter performance is tested 24 hours a day. Ultrasound-guided vascular catheter placement has to be done. The choice of vein in order is as follows, right internal jugular vein > femoral vein. The subclavian and left internal jugular vein has to be avoided.[9,10] The right internal jugular vein gives the best result as there is a pool of blood in the form of right atrium which helps in a less resistant flow in the catheter. If femoral vein is to be selected, the catheter has to be introduced at least >20 cm in order to avoid recirculation inside the catheter. Using a blood pump, the patient's blood is removed via the red coded line (Access) typically connected to the red port of the catheter and delivered through the hemofilter back to the patient via the blue coded line (Return) typically connected to the blue port.[11]

## Anticoagulation

Anticoagulants are used to prevent the blood from clotting within the extracorporeal circuit during the CRRT procedure. CRRT uses various anticoagulants; the most common of them are heparin and citrate. Details of anticoagulation are dealt in a separate chapter.

## Fluids

The primary function of fluids (dialysate/replacement) is to facilitate removal of solutes via diffusion or convection. These fluids do not affect the patient's intravascular volume.

## Blood Warmers

Hypothermia may occur during CRRT as a result of prolonged blood circulation in an extracorporeal circuit. Hence blood warmers or external warming devices are recommended to prevent hypothermia.

## WHAT DOSE?

It has to be understood that the dosage of CRRT is completely different from that of IHD.[3] Whereas in IHD, KT/V (UREA) is considered to be the dosing option; the same is not true for patients who are critically ill. These patients are having a variable volume of distribution, they are metabolically unstable, frequently on vasopressors, are having some residual kidney function left, making them completely different from relatively stable patients where IHD is an option. In CRRT, the *dose* is calculated on the basis of the *rate of effluent volume.*

In the earlier part of this century, many users were in an opinion to use a higher dose (40 mL/kg/hr) of effluent volume which was found to have mortality benefit over lower doses (25 mL/kg/hr.). However this was challenged by two large trials, one from the USA (ATN) and the other from Australia (RENAL) which showed that higher effluent volume does not have any mortality benefit over lower effluent volumes. Though researchers have found that higher dosage might be useful in reversing the vasopressor use in septic shock, the *general consensus is to use a dose of 25 mL/kg/hr of effluent volume.* However, *the prescribed dose should be higher* as there might be multiple stoppage times affecting the dosage (DOREMI).[4] *So in order to achieve the recommended dose you have to prescribe a higher dose.*

*The recommendation is*:

1. Effluent volume of 25 mL/kg/hr is the recommended dose (KDIGO 2012)[1]
2. Prescribe a higher dose to achieve this dose
3. Dosage must be individualized according to patient needs.

## INDICATIONS OF CRRT

Continuous renal replacement therapy has found its use mainly in the intensive care where *hemodynamically and metabolically unstable* critically ill patients suffering from *acute kidney injury (AKI)* are treated. Continuous therapy being slow, avoids rapid intercompartmental shifts and thus obviating hypotension and disequilibrium syndromes frequently seen with intermittent therapies. They have *excellent volume control* and *correct metabolic acidosis* and *severe electrolyte disturbances*. They also remove excess of fluids from the patient and this helps significantly to improve *cerebral edema* and *diuretic resistant hypotensive pulmonary edema*. The process causes hypothermia, one of its side effects which can be utilized judiciously in patients of *malignant hyperthermia*. Its ability to remove middle molecules which are responsible for the pathogenesis of sepsis, makes it an attractive choice in patients of sepsis as an adjuvant therapy. However the theoretical advantage has not yet been reflected in randomized control trials. Its advantage over intermittent therapies in renal recovery, as shown by different observational studies and meta-analysis, makes it a favorite to treat critically ill patients with acute kidney injuries. Finally patients of AKI and acute respiratory distress syndrome (ARDS) have a high incidence of mortality. CRRT can be judiciously used in these situations to remove carbon dioxide by attaching a neonatal oxygenator in the circuit. This process of *extracorporeal carbon dioxide removal (ECCO2R)* helps in achieving very low tidal volume (3 mL/kg—XTRAVENT Study).[5] This also helps in obviating *permissive hypercapnia*, which used to highlight the inability of the intensivists to remove the excess of carbon dioxide and thus had no other choice but to permit the evil hypercapnia to thrive. It has also entered the liver transplant intensive care to be used as a bridge therapy in patients of *acute liver failure*. Thus in short, CRRT has a host of *renal and nonrenal indications* in critically ill patients making its horizon wider as an instrument of *renal support* rather than a simple therapy (Table 1).

## WHEN TO START?

Consensus regarding as to when to start CRRT is yet to be achieved. Most of the earlier studies in the initial part of the decade were in favor of early start of therapy. However the criteria of early therapy were vague. The Risk, Injury, Failure, Loss, End-Stage (RIFLE)[12], Acute Kidney Injury Network (AKIN)[13], and Kidney Disease Improving Global Outcomes (KDIGO) classifications have helped in classifying AKI according to the increasing order of severity.[1] The recent trials of Artificial Kidney Initiation in Kidney Injury (AKIKI)[14] and Early Versus Late Initiation of Renal Replacement Therapy In Critically Ill Patients With Acute Kidney Injury (ELAIN)[15] have contradictory results. The general consensus is to individualize patients and start CRRT accordingly.

**Table 1:** Indications of CRRT

| *Renal indications* | *Nonrenal indications* |
|---|---|
| • Rapidly worsening acute kidney injury (AKI) | • Malignant hyperthermia |
| • Rapidly worsening illness severity along with AKI | • Diuretic resistant pulmonary edema |
| • Reduced renal reserve | • Acute liver failure |
| • Low probability of renal recovery | • Cerebral edema |
| | • Permissive hypercapnia (ECCO2R) |
| | • Electrolyte imbalances |
| | • Tumor lysis syndrome |
| | • Selected toxins |
| | • Hypercatabolic states, severe sepsis |

## WHEN TO STOP?

*As Per KDIGO 2012,* RRT is discontinued when it is no longer required, either because intrinsic kidney function has recovered to the point that it is adequate to meet patient needs, or because RRT is no longer consistent with the goals of care. However, it should be made sure that the patient is in optimal condition (hemodynamics, volume and electrolyte status, metabolic status) before RRT is terminated. Abrupt stoppage of CRRT is discouraged. It is advisable to shift to conventional intermittent modes till the patient completely regains his/her renal function.

Of late, *protocolized weaning from CRRT* is practiced in many centers. If the patient condition is stable hemodynamically, and his respiratory functions are stable, the probable cause and sequel of AKI has been addressed, and the urine output is >30 mL/hr, then *measure the 24 hour urinary creatinine in the intradialytic period.* ***If*** *the value of urinary creatinine is >5.2 mmol/L, cessation of CRRT could be attempted.*

## PRESCRIBING CRRT

### Choice of Modality (SCUF/CVVHD/CVVH/CVVHDF)

Selection of modality depends on condition of patient, target solutes to be removed, and the course of treatment.

### Delivery of Therapy

A key element of the CRRT delivery is effluent dose. Until recently, little evidence existed for dosing, which led to wide variations in clinical practice. For continuous techniques, dose is the sum of all effluent fluids expressed as milliliters per kilogram body weight per hour. It is important to note that the addition of dialysate and the targeting of negative fluid balance both add to the summative dose.

- The dose of CRRT can be thought of as the volume of blood "purified" per unit time. The treatment dose is usually prescribed as an hourly "exchange rate" which is the desired hourly flow rate adjusted for the patient's weight. More definitively the dose is the clearance rate of a representative marker solute; usually indexed to body weight (K/wt = L/kg/hr).[18,19]

- In clinical practice the "dose" of CRRT is the effluent flow rate (= ultrafiltrate + dialysate)
- The effluent flow rate (Qef) is the final result of the filtration process and is composed of the net ultrafiltration (Qnet) plus substitution fluid rate (Qs) in CVVH and CVVHDF plus dialysate flow rate in CVVHD and CVVHDF.[7,18,19]
- Effluent volumes of 20–25 mL/Kg/hr are currently considered to be sufficient with little evidence to support higher dosages.
- Delivered dosages are often less than prescribed dosages due to predilution and down time. In clinical practice to achieve delivered dose of 20–25 mL/kg/hr, prescription should be in the range of 30–35 mL/kg/hr.
- In the case of CVVH, the exchange rate simply represents the ultrafiltration rate whereas in CVVHDF it represents a combination of the ultrafiltration rate and the dialysate flow rate.

## Setting Flow Rates

### *Blood Flow Rate*

Blood flow rates should be optimized to reduce filter clotting and improve efficiency.

In order to maximize small molecule clearance and minimize filter clotting:[16]

- *For continuous hemodialysis: Qb ≥ 2–2.5 × Qd*
- *For post filter continuous hemofiltration: Qb ≥ 5 × Qr*
- *For pre filter continuous hemofiltration: Qb ≥ 6 × Qr*

*Example:*

- *For CVVHD* with Qd 2,000 mL/hr (33 mL/min): Qb ≥ 83 mL/min
- *For post filter CVVHF* with Qr 2,000 mL/hr (33 mL/min): Qb ≥ 165 mL/min
- *For pre filter CVVHDF* with Qr 1,000 mL/hr (17 mL/min) and Qd 1,500 mL/hr (25 mL/min): Qb ≥ 100 mL/min (i.e. the larger of 17 × 6 = 100 or 25 × 2.5 = 63)

### *Dialysate and Replacement Rates*

*Depending on the modality used, dialysate or replacement rates can typically range between 17 mL/min and 33 mL/min in CRRT.*

The decision to infuse *replacement fluids* before or after the filter is made by the physician. *Replacement fluids* administered pre filter reduce filter clotting and can be administered at faster rates (driving higher *convection*) than fluids administered post filter. *The downside of pre filter replacement fluids is that they reduce effective clearance up to 10–15%.* But on the contrary, postdilution replacement fluids may not reduce clearance but limits UF rates due to hemoconcentration of blood.[17] Hence replacement fluids should be infused as a pre and postdilution split to maximize both filter life (predilution) and solute clearance (postdilution). *Many clinicians prefer to infuse predilution and postdilution fluid in the ration of 1/3:2/3rd.*

In CVVHDF, the ratio of ultrafiltration to dialysate flow is often set at 1:1 but it can be altered to put the emphasis on either the dialysis or filtration component.

## Patient Fluid Removal

Fluid removed directly from the patient's intravascular compartment. Hourly rate of removal is prescribed by the physician. Non-CRRT intakes and outputs must be calculated and considered.

*Considerations for mechanical fluid removal:*[7]

- The total amount of fluid that needs to be removed to achieve clinical goals.
- Ongoing fluid administration needs as well as ongoing net inputs and outputs
- Hemodynamic status (blood pressure, need for ongoing pressor support)
- Rate at which fluid needs to be removed from the patient
- Need for solute removal, electrolyte correction or control of uremia.

*Patient fluid removal rate (to be set on machine) = Net fluid removal (hrly) + Non-CRRT intake - Non-CRRT output*[7]

*Example:*

- Mr X is a 50-year-old male on CRRT-CVVHDF day 3. The intensivist set order for fluid as is 100 mL/hr based on previous day I/O balance. In the last hour, the patient has received 200 mL of tube feeds, he has also received IV vancomycin at the rate of 100 mL/hr. His last hour drain output was 50 mL and urine output 120 mL. Calculate the patient fluid removal rate to be set on the machine.
- Net fluid removal (Intensivist order) = 100 mL
- Non-CRRT intake: 200 (feed) + 100 (injection) = 300 mL
- Non-CRRT output: 50 (drain) + 120 (urine) = 170 mL
- Patient fluid removal to be set in machine = (100 + 300) –170 = 230 mL
- If you set 100 mL in machine, it will be 230 - 100 = 130 mL positive fluid balance!!!!

*Example of setting up a prescription:*

Hence from the above inference in case if we have a patient weighing 80 kg prescribed for CRRT-CVVHDF modality. Following may be the prescription:

*In CVVHDF, Qeff = Qr + Qd + Qpfr*

Where Qeff = effluent rate,

Qr = replacement rate (pre filter+ post filter)

Qd = dialysate rate

Qpfr = patient fluid removal rate

If Qpfr = 0, *then Qeff = Qd + Qr* and is called *zero balanced CRRT*

If Qpfr is +ve, *then Qeff > Qd + Qr* and is called *negative balanced CRRT*

Current CRRT machines like Prismaflex only allow zero balanced and negative balanced CRRT but not positive balanced CRRT.

*Example:*

- *CVVHDF*:
  - Total dose = Effluent rate = DR + UFR
  - Total dose = DR + RFR

*Example:*

- ◆ Dialysate rate = 1,000 mL/hr
- ◆ Ultrafiltrate rate (replacement fluid) = 1,000 mL/hr
- ◆ Effluent rate = 1,000 + 1,000 = 2,000 mL/hr
- ◆ In a 50 kg individual, EFR = 2,000/50 = 40 mL/kg/hr

- Dialysate rate + UFR rate = effluent rate = *Zero Balanced*
- Patient fluid removal = 100 mL/hr
- EFR = 1,000 + 1,000 + 100 = 2,100 = 2,100/50 = 42 mL/kg/hr
- If PFR is added then *EF>DR+ UFR= Negative balanced*

- *SCUF*:
  - *Dialysate Rate(0) + UF (0) + PFR 100 mL/hr = SCUF*
- *CVVHD*:
  - Dialysate rate = 1,000 mL/hr
  - Ultrafiltrate rate (replacement fluid) = 0 mL/hr
  - Effluent rate = 1,000 mL/hr + 0 = 1,000 mL/hr
  - In a 50 kg individual, EFR = 1,000/50 = 20 mL/kg/hr
- *CVVHF*:
  - Dialysate rate = 0
  - Ultrafiltrate rate (replacement fluid) = 1,000 mL/hr
  - Effluent rate = 0 + 1,000 = 1,000 mL/hr
  - In a 50 kg individual, EFR = 1,000/50 = 20 mL/kg/hr

  It has already been mentioned that the prescribed clearance is always more than the actual clearance. The clearance is also affected by predilution, which decreases the clearance. This is explained by the following example.

  - Pre filter replacement QRF = 300 mL/hr
  - Dialysate rate QD = 1,000 mL/hr
  - Fluid removal rate QRR = 700 mL/hr
  - Effluent rate QE = 300 + 1000 + 700 = 2,000 mL/hr
  - *Prescribed dose= 2,000/50 mL/kg/hr = 40 mL/kg/hr*
  - Blood flow = 100 mL/min = 100 × 60 = 6,000 mL/hr
  - QBW = *Blood Water Flow Rate* =(1 – HCT) × Blood flow mL/hr
  - Blood water flow QBW = (1 – 0.3 ) × 6,000 mL/hr = 0.7 × 6000 = 4,200 mL/hr
  - *Effective dose:*

    = QE [(QBW/QBW + QRF)]/W mL/kg/hr

    = 2,000 [4,200/4,200 + 300]/50

    = 2,000 × (4,200/4,500)/50

    = *37 mL/kg/hr*
  - Actual total effluent volume = *1,600 mL (Less Due to Stoppage Times)*

    Actual dose = 1,600 × (4,200/4,500)/50 = 29 mL/kg/hr

## Setting Anticoagulation Rates

Some form of anticoagulation is generally preferred to maintain filter patency unless contraindicated.

Unfractionated heparin: 5–10 IU/kg/hr

Citrate: 3 mmol/L blood

Once all the flow parameters are entered, the treatment is started and patient is monitored. Parameters can be titered later in case needed during the treatment. A successful CRRT therapy would aim to ensure complete benefits to the patients by minimizing interruptions in the treatment and reducing downtime.

The final prescription will look something like this:

1. Type of therapy : CVVHF/CVVHD/CVVHDF
2. Filter : AN69 M100
3. Blood flow : 140 mL/min
4. Predilution : 300 mL/hr
5. Postdilution/replacement : 700 mL/hr
6. Dialysate : 1,000 mL/hr
7. Patient fluid removal : 230 mL/hr
8. Anticoagulation : Heparin/citrate/none
9. Anticoagulation Dose : Heparin—5 IU/kg/hr; Citrate—3 mmol/L blood
10. Effluent rate : 40 mL/kg/hr
11. Effective dose : 37 mL/kg/hr
12. Zero balanced/negative balanced
13. Standard additives: Potassium and phosphate, e.g. Add KCl 40 mEq/5L bag if serum potassium <4 mmol/l. Needs phosphate replacement if <1 mmol/L (60 mmol/day)

## SUMMARY

Continuous renal replacement therapy is a therapy that is gaining greater acceptance and becoming more widely used for treatment of both renal and nonrenal indications. And in the population of critically ill patients, CRRT is one of the best RRT options these hemodynamically unstable patients may tolerate. A physician and critical care nurse/technician plays a very important role through setting up the right prescription, continuous monitoring, and identification of any problems and resolving it at the earliest for the successful running of therapy.

## REFERENCES

1. Kidney Disease Improving Global Outcomes (KDIGO) Acute Kidney Injury Work Group. KDIGO clinical practice guideline for acute kidney injury. Kidney Int Suppl. 2012.
2. Palevsky PM, Zhang JH, O'Connor TZ, et al; VA/NIH Acute Renal Failure Trial Network. Intensity of renal support in critically ill patients with acute kidney injury. New Engl J Med. 2008;359(1):7-20.

3. Bellomo R, Cass A, Cole L, et al; RENAL Replacement Therapy Study Investigators. Intensity of continuous renal-replacement therapy in critically ill patients. New Engl J Med. 2009;361(17):1627-38.
4. Vesconi S, Cruz DN, Fumagalli R, et al. Delivered dose of RRT and mortality in critically ill patients with AKI (DO-RE-MI Study group). Crit Care. 2009;13(2):R57.
5. Bein T, Weber-Carstens S, Goldmann A, et al. Lower tidal volume strategy (≈3 ml/kg) combined with extracorporeal CO2 removal versus 'conventional' protective ventilation (6 ml/kg) in severe ARDS: the prospective randomized Xtravent-study. Intensive Care Med. 2013;39(5):847-56.
6. Mortell M (2006), Prisma workshop, NGHA-CR
7. Prismaflex®8.xx Operators manual 2015
8. Gambro self learning module – CRRT, 2010
9. Ronco C, Bellomo R, LaGreca, (Eds): Blood Purification in Intensive Care. Contrib Nephrol. Basel, Karger, vol 132, pp 266-82.
10. CRRT learning package, NSW health, Intensive Care Unit.
11. CRRT Overview- Module1, Critical care Nephrology alliance, 2007.
12. Bellomo R, RoncoC, Kellum JA , et al. Palevsky P and the ADQI workgroup. Acute renal failure— definition, outcome measures, animal models, fluid therapy and information technology needs: the Second International Consensus Conference of the Acute Dialysis Quality Initiative (ADQI) Group, Crit Care , 2004, vol. 8 pg. R204.
13. Mehta RL, Kellum JA, Shah SV, et al. Acute Kidney Injury Network: report of an initiative to improve outcomes in acute kidney injury, Crit Care , 2007, vol. 11 pg. R31.
14. AKIKI. Gaudry et al. NEJM 2016; 375:122-33.
15. ELAIN. Zarbock. JAMA 2016; 315(20):2190-99.
16. Sambandam K; Hamdi, T. ASN innovations in Kidney education- CRRT simulator powerpoint.
17. https://www.slideshare.net/samirelansary/crrt-2-45953506.
18. https://lifeinthefastlane.com/ccc/renal-replacement-therapy-prescription/
19. https://nephrology.hosted.panopto.com/Panopto/Pages/Viewer.aspx?id=a16e55fa-e8c7-487c-be40-a931010932d7.

CHAPTER 9

# Set Up and Prescription for Sustained Low-efficiency Dialysis

*Sunil Karanth*

## INTRODUCTION

Acute kidney injury (AKI) is a common and important problem occurring in many patients in an intensive care unit (ICU). The incidence varies from 5.7% to 19% in different populations studied.[1] The concern with the development of AKI, is the doubling of mortality in patients with AKI to as high as 52%. Over the years, multiple modalities of renal replacement therapies (RRTs) have emerged for the management of AKI patients, especially when they are critically ill. Starting from the early primitive dialysis by Dr WJ Kollef to the modification incorporated in the Alwall dialyzer, intermittent hemodialysis (IHD) from a technological and clinical perspective has come a long way. Newer modalities of therapy like continuous renal replacement therapy (CRRT), was developed, as early as 1960, and from then to now has evolved as one of the mainstay methods of RRT.[2] Despite the developments, there are numerous pros and cons in both the well-established modalities, when they are applied in the clinical context.

The advantages of IHD are that it provides the required dialysis dose in a short period of time (giving time for other therapies and patient movements for various procedures), is economical, needing less manpower, and provides good solute clearance by using diffusion as the physical principle of clearance. The disadvantages of IHD are its practical lack of applicability in hemodynamically unstable patients, lack of middle molecule clearance due to absence of convection and need for having supply of pure Reverse Osmosis (RO) water for provision of dialysis.

Continuous renal replacement therapy on the other hand, has the advantage of providing RRT in hemodynamically unstable patients, with excellent middle molecule clearance and can be provided in patient areas where the RO water supply does not exist. But CRRT has the disadvantage of high cost, is labor intensive, limited solute clearance, and need for disconnections when various clinical cares need to be provided (reducing the total dose of dialysis in a 24-hour period).

Hence a need was felt for development of a hybrid technique of RRT which could have the advantages of IHD and RRT combined, minimizing the negative aspects of these two forms. This hybrid technique developed was called sustained low-efficiency daily dialysis.[3] Sustained low-efficiency daily dialysis was first introduced about two decades ago. It provides RRT at a dialysate rate of 100–300 mL/min and a blood flow rate of 100–200 mL/min for a prolonged period (6–12 hours) using a high-flux or low-flux dialyzer or hemofilter. Similar to CRRT, the lack of hour to hour clearance is compensated by extending the duration of therapy. The lower blood flow and dialysate flow rate provide for better hemodynamic tolerance and a reduced risk of dialysis disequilibrium, making it feasible to be used in critically ill, hemodynamically unstable patients. Besides, as the therapy is not continuous (like CRRT), it provides substantial time-off periods for other cares reducing the chances of dialysis disconnections. This makes it less labor intensive and more pragmatic to be used in the ICU setting. However, sustained low-efficiency daily dialysis still carries the disadvantage of needing RO water supply at the site of provision of care.

In recent times, sustained low-efficiency daily dialysis can be provided by most machines able to offer IHD, as the newer generation machines are able to provide and monitor lower flow states. The dialysate fluid used has the same composition as the ones used for IHD. However, in view of the prolonged duration of the treatment, it is important to intermittently monitor electrolyte levels, especially serum potassium levels as would be done in the case of CRRT. The ultrafiltration can be pre-set as per the need, taking into account the patient's fluid balance, hemodynamic status, and the infusions given during the hours of dialysis. Intradialytic therapy adjustments can be further made to the ultrafiltration targets based on the patient's clinical state. The newer generation machines also provide addition of the convective process of hemofiltration as well, called sustained low-efficiency daily dialysis-f. Principles of anticoagulation remain as for any other modality of RRT. This ranges from the time-tested heparin infusion to citrate to no anticoagulation when the risks of anticoagulation far outweigh the risk of clotting of the circuit.

## SET UP AND COMMENCEMENT OF SUSTAINED LOW-EFFICIENCY DAILY DIALYSIS

Since this is meant to be a clinical guide, the steps of setting up the sustained low-efficiency daily dialysis will largely be restricted to the clinical management aspects on this subject. A detailed technical description of the setting up of machine can be obtained from the manual of the respective machines.

- Decision is made to provide RRT in the form of sustained low-efficiency daily dialysis.
- Inform the nephrology team and the dialysis technician to set up the machine.
- Ensure a good vascular access is available to initiate RRT.
- Machine to go through all the relevant checks.
- Set up the Dialysis Delivery System.
- Prepare the extracorporeal blood circuit.
- Conduct pressure and alarm tests.
- Plan goals of therapy:
  - Sustained low-efficiency daily dialysis/Sustained low-efficiency daily dialysis-f
  - *Blood flow*: Start at 100–150 mL/min. If the patient is stable on initiation of therapy, increase to higher flow rates as required.
  - *Dialysate rate*: Start at 100–150 mL/min if patient is extremely unstable or higher (up to 300 mL/min) for severe acidosis or hyperkalemia (100 mL/min is the lowest available on

the 5008 and NCU 18 machines, and 200 on Dialog plus. All the others have a lower limit of 300 mL/min.)

- *Ultrafiltration goal*: It is based on hemodynamic tolerance and the clinical need. Remember to factor in the volume of infusions likely to be administered as medications and other therapies during the duration of the RRT.
- *Duration of therapy*:
  - 6 hours
  - 8 hours
  - 12 hours
  - Extend as needed.
- *Assess regarding the need for anticoagulation*:
  - Rule out contraindications for anticoagulation
  - Decide on need and dose of priming the circuit with heparin (generally 1,000 units of heparin used for priming the circuit).
  - Assess the pros and cons of heparin anticoagulation:
    - Bolus dosing—necessity, safety, and dosing
    - Infusion—necessity, safety, and dosing
    - Activated partial thromboplastin time (APTT) targets—generally as in CRRT the goal is to keep the target between 45 seconds and 60 seconds.
  - Watch for risk of nonbleeding complications of heparin like heparin-induced thrombocytopenia
  - Assess for alternative forms of anticoagulation: Studies are available to indicate that regional citrate anticoagulation is a good alternative to systemic anticoagulation. 30% citrate as an infusion in the arterial side of the catheter may be a good clinical alternative.[4]
- *Dialysate fluid options*: Generally, the standard dialysate fluid used for IHD can be selected. The standard settings on the sustained low-efficiency daily dialysis would be:
  - Sodium conductance of 140 (unless dealing with a patient with long-standing hyponatremia, wherein a lower sodium concentration is used).
  - Dialysate solutions with a potassium concentration of 2.5 or 3 mmol/L. The choice of fluid will be based on the pretreatment potassium values. It is important to monitor the potassium levels at least once after 3–4 hours of therapy to avoid life-threatening hypokalemia, as sustained low-efficiency daily dialysis is a form of prolonged RRT with a risk of significant electrolyte disturbances.
  - Bicarbonate settings: To begin with, default settings of 35–37 mmol/L will be used and maintained throughout the therapy, unless the patient is alkalotic when a lower level is set on the machine.
- *Monitoring of therapy*:
  - Monitoring of the critically ill patient:
    - Hemodynamic monitoring, if need be by invasive or semi-invasive methods
    - Monitoring of other systemic parameters like central nervous system and respiratory system

- ◊ Monitoring other organ supports whenever provided, such as mechanical ventilation, cardiovascular support, etc.
- Monitoring specifically with respect to sustained low-efficiency daily dialysis:
  - ◊ Arterial blood gas (ABG) at least by 3–4 hours of therapy to assess:
    - Response to RRT—clearance/correction of acidosis
    - Serum potassium levels
  - ◊ In patients on sustained low-efficiency daily dialysis for many days:
    - Monitoring of other electrolytes like serum magnesium and serum phosphate on a periodic basis is necessary.

## SUSTAINED LOW-EFFICIENCY DAILY DIALYSIS VERSUS OTHER MODALITIES OF RRT IN THE ICU

Sustained low-efficiency daily dialysis is certainly found to be superior to IHD in terms of better hemodynamic stability as compared to the latter.[5] In a meta-analysis,[6] Zhang et al. found that sustained low-efficiency daily dialysis was equivalent to CRRT in terms of recovery of renal function, days of stay in the ICU, and biochemical clearance. In fact, the analysis favored sustained low-efficiency daily dialysis compared to CRRT in terms of mortality. But this result was largely based on observational studies as the analysis included 10 observational studies and 7 randomized controlled trials. Hence larger, multicentric studies may be needed to prove the superiority of sustained low-efficiency daily dialysis over CRRT. But certainly, the literature points toward equivalence between sustained low-efficiency daily dialysis and CRRT in most of the outcomes measured.

## CONCLUSION

Sustained low-efficiency daily dialysis is a hybrid modality of RRT evolved over the last two decades, trying to combine the benefits of IHD and CRRT. Sustained low-efficiency daily dialysis seems to provide clinical benefits similar to CRRT, at a more economical cost and less labor intensive too. More studies are essential to ascertain if sustained low-efficiency daily dialysis is superior than CRRT as a mode of RRT in the ICU, as current literature largely show both modalities to be equally efficacious.

### SUSTAINED LOW-EFFICIENCY DAILY DIALYSIS PRESCRIPTION FORM

1. **Notify Dialysis Unit to initiated SLED**
2. **Diagnostics:**
   - ☐ PTT now
   - ☐ Platelet count
   - ☐ Hb
   - ☐ Other: ______________________________
3. **Assessments:**
   Hourly vital signs and SLED parameters per flowsheet
   Weigh patient pre- and post-SLED (if possible)

**4. Notify physician if:**

☐ Vasopressors need to be increased to maintain SLED at ordered settings

☐ SBP is less than or equal to _______ or MAP is less than or equal to _________

☐ Other: _______

5. ______ **Machine:**

Treatment time: ☐ 8 hrs ☐ 12 hrs ☐ Other _____ hrs (document reason in progress note)

Fluid removal goal: ☐ Maintain neutral balance during SLED ☐ Remove _____ mL/hr

☐ Net removal ______ mL

Use vascular access:______________________________

Blood flow rate (usually 200–250 mL/min): ☐ 200 mL/min ☐ Other:_____ mL/min

Dialysate flow rate (max. 300 mL/min): ☐ 100 mL/min ☐ Other:_____ mL/min

☐ May be adjusted by SLED nurse

Dialyzer: ________

Dialysate:

Sodium: _________mEq

Bicarbonate: ☐ 35 mEq ☐ 30 mEq ☐ Other:_____ mEq

Potassium: ☐ 2 mEq ☐ 3 mEq ☐ 3.5 mEq

☐ Other:_____ mEq

Calcium: ☐ 2 mEq ☐ 3 mEq ☐ 3.5 mEq

☐ Other:_____ mEq

**6. Medications:**

Consult clinical pharmacist for dosing and timing of antibiotics during treatment

☐ No heparin

☐ Prime circuit with 1,000 units of heparin

- ☐ Give prime
- ☐ Waste prime

☐ Bolus with heparin _______ units at the initiation of SLED

☐ Heparin 25,000 units in 500 mL D5W infusion at_____ units/hr during SLED treatment

**7. PRN Volume Expanders during SLED:**

☐ Normal saline 100–200 mL IV

☐ May repeat x _____ doses

☐ May repeat as needed

☐ Mannitol 12.5 g/50 mL ☐ ☐ ☐ ☐ at start of treatment

☐ q 1 hr x _____ doses

☐ ☐ ☐ Albumin 25%, 12.5 g IV ☐ ☐ at start of treatment

☐ q 1 hr x _____ doses

## REFERENCES

1. Uchino S, Kellum JA, Bellomo R, et al. Acute renal failure in critically ill patients: a multinational, multicenter study. JAMA. 2005;294:813-8.
2. Fleming GM. Renal replacement therapy review. Organogenesis. 2011;7:1:2-12.
3. Kumar V, Craig M, Depner T, et al. Extended daily dialysis: a new approach to renal replacement therapy for acute renal failure in the intensive care unit. Am J Kidney Dis. 2000;36:294-300.
4. Wen M, Küchle C, Steubl D, et al. A novel citrate-based protocol versus heparin anticoagulation for sustained low efficiency dialysis in the ICU: safety, efficacy, and cost. BMC Nephrol. 2018;19:79.
5. Cornelis T, van der Sande FM, Eloot S, et al. Acute hemodynamic response and uremic toxin removal in conventional and extended hemodialysis and hemodiafiltration: a randomized crossover study. Am J Kidney Dis. 2014;64:247-56.
6. Zhang L, Yang J, Eastwood GM, et al. Extended daily dialysis versus continuous renal replacement therapy for acute kidney injury: a meta-analysis. Am J Kidney Dis. 2015;66:322-30.

CHAPTER 10

# Anticoagulation on RRT

*Pradeep D'costa*

## INTRODUCTION

Critically ill patients with acute kidney injury (AKI) requiring dialysis form a sizeable proportion of the seriously ill patients we encounter in the ICU. Dialysis of these patients is sometimes a very challenging task and requires close monitoring.

One of the main preconditions for performing a smooth dialysis is maintaining the patency of the extracorporeal circuit (ECC). During renal replacement therapy (RRT), blood comes in contact with ECC including the catheter, dialyzer or hemofilter, and blood tubings, i.e. "nonphysiological environments" all of which could activate the coagulation pathways, leading to clotting. Also in AKI in ICU, disruption of procoagulant-anticoagulant system balance in favor of increase in the procoagulant state secondary to endothelial cell activation and upregulation of thrombospondin is seen. Clotting leads to reduced dialysis efficiency, reduced circuit lifespan, increased manpower usage, increased blood loss, increased consumption of materials, and hence costs of treatment.

The benefits of anticoagulation to achieve adequate RRT by preventing filter clotting have to be weighed against the risk of bleeding, resource availability, and cost issues. A subtle balance between under and over anticoagulation requires to be maintained to prevent complications from developing. This article discusses some points that can be considered for treating such patients.

## FACTORS ASSOCIATED WITH INCREASED CLOTTING ON ECC

Exposure of blood to ECC components leads to release of contact activation factors triggering intrinsic pathway of coagulation. This process is exacerbated by different factors as below:

- Kinks in catheters, tubings associated with turbulence
- Catheter factors like insertion site, tip position, side holes, length and internal diameter
- Dialysis access recirculation
- Dialyzer membrane characteristics (high negative charge associated with higher clotting)
- Pumped versus nonpumped systems (e.g. CAVH)
- Low blood flow rates
- High ultrafiltration rate contributing to hemoconcentration

- Predilution versus postdilution replacement (effect of viscosity)
- High hematocrit of patient
- Air-blood interface: Volume of air traps, retained air in dialyzer, due to inadequate priming
- Intradialytic blood, blood products, albumin and lipid infusion
- Patient/disease factors like prothrombotic state.

## IDENTIFYING CLOTTING IN THE EXTRACORPOREAL CIRCUIT[1]

The signs of clotting in the ECC are:

- Extremely dark blood
- Shadows or black streaks in the dialyzer
- Foaming with subsequent clot formation in drip chambers and venous trap
- Rapid filling of transducer monitors with blood
- "Tethering" (blood in the postdialyzer venous line segment that is unable to continue into the venous chamber but falls back into the line segment)
- Presence of clots at the arterial side header
- Increase in ECC pressures depending upon the site of clotting.

## AVAILABLE OPTIONS FOR ANTICOAGULATION

Ideal anticoagulation for ECC should be effective, cheap, safe with low bleeding risks, easily monitored, and reversible, if required. Choice of anticoagulants in clinical practice is based on various factors like availability of drug, costs, and available modalities of monitoring in addition to patient factors. Table 1 describes various methods of anticoagulation used in different clinical scenarios.

Among all the available anticoagulants, unfractionated heparin (UFH) is the most widely used worldwide, as anticoagulant, due to following reasons:

- Widespread availability
- Low costs
- Relative ease of use.

**Table 1:** Anticoagulation methods on dialysis.

| *Heparin-related anticoagulation* | *Citrate-related anticoagulation* | *Heparin/ anticoagulant free dialysis* | *Others* |
|---|---|---|---|
| Unfractionated heparin (UFH) | Regional citrate anticoagulation | No saline flushes | Heparinoids: heparin mixtures, direct thrombin inhibitors |
| Low molecular weight heparin (LMWH) | Bicarbonate dialysate with low concentration citrate: Citrasate | Saline flushes: intermittent saline flushes vs. continuous saline infusion | Prostacyclin |
| Regional heparinization with protamine reversal | | | Serine protease inhibitors: Nafamostat mesilate, Aprotinin |
| Heparin coated dialyzer filters | | | |

Today worldwide, regional citrate anticoagulation (RCA) is recommended as the anticoagulation of choice for the majority of critically ill patients requiring continuous renal replacement therapy (CRRT)/sustained low-efficiency dialysis (SLED) today. Since these patients are at increased risk of bleeding, RCA is preferred over no anticoagulation/other systemic anticoagulation because of the regional nature of anticoagulation with citrate with no to minimal risk of systemic bleeding when monitored appropriately.

Table 2 summarizes the mechanism of action, monitoring strategy, advantages, and drawbacks of the common anticoagulants used during RRT in the intensive care setting.

**Table 2:** Various anticoagulants and their salient features.[2]

| *Agent* | *Half-life* | *Dose* | *Monitoring* | *Antidote* | *Remarks* |
|---|---|---|---|---|---|
| Unfractionated heparin | 60 minutes increased to 180 in AKI | Loading 10–20 U/kg, then 3–12 U/kg/hr | ACT = 120–180 sec<br>aPTT = 35–45 sec prefilter | Protamine 1 mg/100 units | • Hypotension and HIT II possible<br>• Nondialyzable |
| Regional heparinization | - | Loading 5–10 U/kg then 3–12 U/kg/hr with protamine 1 mg/100 units | aPTT = 100–140 sec prefilter, systemic normal | - | • Nondialyzable |
| LMWH | • Enoxaparin 24 hours<br>• Tinzaparin 5 hours | • IHD Enoxaparin 0.8–1 mg/kg<br>• Tinzaparin 3,500 units<br>• CRRT Dalteparin 600 units/hr<br>• Tinzaparin 400–800 U/hr | Anti-Xa, if available | • Protamine may be used<br>• It reverses only Anti-Xa activity | • Severe bleeding possible<br>• HIT incidence less as compared to UFH<br>• Nondialyzable |
| Danaparoid | 30 hours | IHD 2,500–3,750 U followed by 2,000–2,500 U/hr | Anti-Xa activity, if available, 0.2–0.4 U/mL | FFP, activated Factor VII required in severe cases | • Increased bleeding risk<br>• Can be used in HIT<br>• Dialyzable |
| Fondaparinux | 17–21 hours | IHD or SLEDD 1.5–2.5 mg | Anti-Xa if available, 0.2–0.4 U/mL | • FFP, activated<br>• Factor VII required in severe cases | • Increased bleeding risk<br>• Can be used in HIT<br>• Dialyzable (high flux or hemofilter) |
| Argatroban | 35 minutes | IHD 0.03 –0.4 mg/kg<br>CRRT 2–2.5 mg/kg | aPTT 2 to 2.5 times normal | • FFP, activated<br>• Factor VII required in severe cases | • Increased bleeding risk<br>• Can be used in HIT<br>• Nondialyzable |
| Prostacyclin | 2 minutes to 2 hours | Titrate from 0.5 ng/kg/min to 2.5–10 ng/kg/min within few minutes of starting treatment | NA | - | • Hypotension<br>• Lack of standard laboratory<br>• Dialyzable |

*Contd...*

*Contd...*

| | | | | | |
|---|---|---|---|---|---|
| Nafamostat mesilate (synthetic serine protease inhibitor) | 5–8 minutes | Priming 20 mg/L NS, then 40 mg/hr | aPTT 1.5 to 2 times normal | No antidote available | • Decreased bleeding risk<br>• Dialyzable |
| Regional citrate anticoagulation | | | Frequent ionized calcium, total calcium estimations Total/Ionized Ca ratio, Acid-base status, lactates, magnesium | _ | • Lack of systemic anticoagulant effect<br>• Preferred in patients at high risk of bleeding<br>• Requires meticulous monitoring |

(ACT: activated clotting time; aPTT: activated partial thromboplastin time; AKI: acute kidney injury; CRRT: continuous renal replacement therapy; FFP: fresh frozen plasma; HIT: heparin-induced thrombocytopenia; IHD: intermittent hemodialysis; LMWH: low molecular weight heparin; SLEDD: sustained low-efficiency daily dialysis; UFH: unfractionated heparin)

## CLOTTING TESTS USED TO MONITOR ANTICOAGULANT THERAPY

Multiple tests for coagulation can be used; however availability of these tests as well as time to obtain results can vary widely from center to center. The type of test depends on the type of anticoagulant used for the dialysis.

The activated partial thromboplastin time (aPTT) and anti-Xa measurements are currently used to monitor UFH and low molecular weight heparin (LMWH) during hemodialysis (HD). During RCA, we need to monitor circuit ionic calcium levels before starting the RCA, at end of first hour, and every 4–6 hours to monitor the anticoagulant effect of citrate.

- The aPTT is used with good accuracy for UFH, but is not adapted for monitoring anticoagulant effect during HD sessions as it requires a delay; its appropriateness for monitoring anticoagulant effect of LMWH during HD is also questionable, so we can use activated clotting time (ACT) which is now available at the bedside in some ICUs, especially coronary care units.
- The determination of anti-Xa activity was used mainly to document attempts to reduce LMWH doses in clinical studies using individualized protocol.
- For more accurate monitoring of coagulation pathways during dialysis, several new biomarkers have been evaluated. Markers like tissue factor pathway inhibitor (TFPI), (soluble) thrombomodulin (TM), and von Willebrand factor (vWF), three biomarkers released from the vascular endothelium; prothrombin fragment 1.2 (F 1.2), and thrombin-antithrombin complex (TAT), two markers of intravascular thrombin generation; plasminogen activator inhibitor-1 (PAI-1), D-dimers, fibrin degradation products; and transforming growth factor-β1 (TGF-β1), a multifunctional cytokine that may act as a mediator of the pleiotropic action of heparin. The predialysis levels of coagulation factors TFPI, TM, and vWF were significantly higher in HD patients than in healthy controls, indicating endothelial dysfunction and a prothrombotic risk. Both UFH and LMWH are potent stimuli of TFPI mobilization. The drawbacks of these tests are the availability and cost.

## OTHER CONSIDERATIONS IN PATIENT ASSESSMENT PRIOR TO COMMENCING ANTICOAGULANT THERAPY

- Patient's fluid status and need for ultrafiltration
- Patient current medication, e.g. anticoagulant, antiplatelet medication
- Patient recent Hb and hematocrit level, WBC
- Anemia treatment
- Medical/surgical history—bleeding/clotting disorders, malignancies
- Pre- or postsurgical intervention
- Previous anticoagulant therapy
- Surface area of dialyzer
- Need for blood product transfusion on dialysis.

## INDIVIDUALIZATION OF ANTICOAGULATION TREATMENT[1,3,4]

The strategy for anticoagulation is individualized to each patient based on the patients' individual risks for developing complications.

- *In patients at high risk of bleeding or pre-existing coagulopathy:*
  - In intermittent RRT or SLED, no anticoagulation should be used (Saline flushes 50–100 mL every 15–30 minutes into prefilter port can be used to maintain circuit patency)
  - In continuous RRT, RCA is preferred to no use of anticoagulation unless there are contraindications to citrate.
- *In patients at low risk of hemorrhage not requiring systemic anticoagulation:*
  - All patients with AKI undergoing RRT should receive anticoagulation if there is no contraindication
  - In intermittent RRT, UFH or LMWH should be preferred to other systemic anticoagulants (with target aPTT 1.5 times the normal)
  - In continuous RRT, RCA is preferred to no use of anticoagulation unless there are contraindications to citrate
  - If citrate anticoagulation is contraindicated or unavailable, UFH (aPTT target 1.5 times the control) is preferred because of its pharmacokinetics and its reversibility compared with LMWH.
- *In patients requiring systemic anticoagulation:*
  - Systemic anticoagulation using UFH should probably be preferred to other anticoagulants
  - In patients on LMWH for deep vein thrombosis (DVT) prophylaxis, use LMWH as single dose at starting RRT.
- *In patients with suspected or proven heparin-induced thrombocytopenia:*
  - Stop heparin administration, both UFH and LMWH
  - Guidelines suggest use of direct thrombin inhibitor (Argatroban) or Factor Xa inhibitors (Fondaparinux, Danaparoid) rather than other or no anticoagulation. Other options: RCA, nafamostat mesilate, or prostacyclin.

Indian guidelines however suggest that UFH should be the anticoagulant of choice during intermittent hemodialysis (IHD) and CRRT when not contraindicated.

## CITRATE ANTICOAGULATION: AN OVERVIEW

Citrate anticoagulation has come up as a safer and much more effective anticoagulation as compared to heparin. Though heparin has been the only available option for anticoagulation for years, it is associated with two main drawbacks:

1. Systemic anticoagulation which is unavoidable.
2. Heparin-induced thrombocytopenia type II (HIT II).

Hence citrate anticoagulation is now the preferred anticoagulation in patients with CRRT (KDIGO 2012). The high probability of clotting of ECC and thereby the need for anticoagulation is high in CRRT as compared to intermittent RRT because of the following reasons:

- Treatment sessions are prolonged
- Blood is pumped through the circuit at a very slow rate
- Underlying prothrombotic state of many of the critically ill patients, e.g. sepsis, trauma.

The major advantage of citrate anticoagulation over heparin is that it is strictly "*Regional*", i.e. anticoagulation is confined to the ECC without any risk of systemic anticoagulation. Hence it is associated with less bleeding, less transfusion, and longer circuit life. In the Indian set up, cost and availability are major limitations. It is also labor intensive. For this reason, in Indian ICUs, UFH still remains the anticoagulant of choice during both intermittent HD and CRRT. In critically ill patients with impaired coagulation like disseminated intravascular coagulation (DIC) or if the bleeding risk is high, IHD and sustained low-efficiency daily dialysis (SLEDD) can be carried out without any anticoagulation.[5]

### Regional Citrate Anticoagulation: Mechanism of Action

It involves administration of citrate which chelates ionized calcium. Calcium is an essential cofactor for generation of thrombin. Anticoagulation is effective when ionized calcium levels fall to below 0.5 mmol/L. Some citrate is cleared as calcium citrate complex through dialysis or filtration. Citrate is metabolized through Krebs cycle in liver, kidneys, and muscles in aerobic conditions. Hence, citrate accumulation and toxicity may be seen in patients with liver diseases and shock. Also, citrate is a buffer base which releases bicarbonate and is administered as sodium salt. This makes it important to have built in protocols in CRRT and also to use dialysate/predilution fluids which are calcium free. The dose of citrate will be titrated on blood flow.

#### *Monitoring of Patients on RCA*

Monitoring requires serial evaluation of:

- Ionized calcium
- Total calcium
- Total/ionized calcium
- Presence of metabolic acidosis and lactates
- As magnesium is also chelated, magnesium levels also need to be monitored.

## *Monitoring Pearls during RCA*

- Decrease in ionized calcium associated with decrease in total calcium indicates inadequate replacement rather than citrate accumulation
- Decrease in ionized calcium with increase in total calcium is associated with citrate accumulation
- Risk of citrate accumulation is high in patients with liver dysfunction and hypoperfusion
- Ratio of total calcium to ionized calcium higher than 2.5 requires temporary stopping of citrate.

Different citrate protocols are available. Use of citrate anticoagulation requires meticulous monitoring and training in protocols.

*Regional citrate anticoagulation use protocol (Courtesy: Dr Valentine Lobo):*

- Prime in continuous venovenous hemodiafiltration (CVVHDF) mode using ordered dialysate and replacement solutions.

  *Dialysate*: $HCO_3$-based without Ca + replacement: Normal saline or bicarb-based industry made solution
- We suggest that regional anticoagulation with Regiocit and Biphozyl may be performed as follows:
  - Set desired blood flow rate
  - Start Regiocit (mL/hr) on the PBP line at 6 times the blood flow rate (e.g. 600 mL/hr for a blood flow of 100 mL/min)
  - Adjust the rate of dialysate and replacement fluid with Biphozyl to obtain an effluent volume of 2L/hr/1.73 $m^2$ or 30 mL/kg/hr
  - Prepare calcium gluconate solution of 250 mL of 10% calcium gluconate with 750 mL 0.9% normal saline
  - Start Ca gluconate infusion (mL/hr) through a separate central line and infusion pump at 0.5 times the blood flow (e.g. 50 mL/hr for a blood flow of 100 mL/hr)
  - Monitor ionic calcium potassium and pH from the blood and ionic calcium from the circuit every 4 hours and adjust infusion rates as per Table 3.

**Table 3:** Patient/circuit ionic calcium levels and citrate dose adjustment.

| | *Citrate dose adjustment for anticoagulant efficiency* | |
|---|---|---|
| Circuit ionic calcium | >20 kg | <20 kg |
| <0.35 | Decrease by 40 mL/hr | Decrease by 20 mL/hr |
| 0.35 to 0.5 | No change | No change |
| 0.5–0.6 | Increase by 40 mL/hr | Increase by 20 mL/hr |
| >0.6 | Increase by 80 mL/hr | Increase by 40 mL/hr |
| Patient ionic calcium | Calcium dose adjustment | |
| >1.3 | Decrease by 10 mL/hr | Decrease by 5 mL/hr |
| 1.1–1.3 | No change | No change |
| 0.9–1.1 | Increase by 10 mL/hr | Increase by 5 mL/hr |
| <0.9 | Increase by 20 mL/hr | Increase by 10 mL/hr |

## NONANTICOAGULANT MEASURES TO REDUCE CIRCUIT AND ACCESS CLOTTING

### Catheter

- *Catheter site*: Right internal jugular, femoral access preferred to left internal jugular and subclavian due to straight course. Do not use femoral catheter in patients with raised intra-abdominal pressures.
- *Catheter tip location*: Femoral catheter tip in inferior vena cava, internal jugular vein tip in right atrium.
- *Catheter length*: Appropriate length (Femoral—20 cm or above), internal diameter and side ports.
- *Catheter type*: Side hole catheters associated with higher recirculation. Shot gun tip catheter preferred.
- Catheter kinking should be avoided.

### Dialysis Mode

- Hemodialysis, hemofiltration with low filtration rate to avoid hemoconcentration
- Predilution hemofiltration
- Avoid low flow rates (<100 mL/min).

## SUMMARY

Clotting on ECC is a major concern as it is associated with decreased efficiency, increased costs/workload, and increased blood transfusions. Balance between anticoagulation and bleeding risk has to be established individually for patients. In patients with minimal bleeding risk, UFH is established anticoagulant therapy. Alternatives like low molecular heparin and heparinoids are not preferred due to monitoring constraints. In patients with high risk of bleeding or contraindication for systemic anticoagulation, regional anticoagulation is preferred. Citrate anticoagulation is recommended over regional UFG–Protamine protocol. RCA requires meticulous protocol for monitoring citrate accumulation and toxicity.

## REFERENCES

1. Indian Journal of Nephrology. (2012). Indian Society of Nephrology Guidelines for Hemodialysis Units. Available from *http://isn-india.org/images/Image/Docs/HD_GL.pdf* [Last Accessed June 2019].
2. Nongnuch A, Tangsujaritvijit V, Davenport A. Anticoagulation for renal replacement therapy for patients with acute kidney injury. Minerva Urol Nefrol. 2016;68(1):87-104.
3. Kidney Disease Improving Global Outcomes (KDIGO) Acute Kidney Injury Work Group. KDIGO clinical practice guideline for acute kidney injury. Kidney Int Suppl. 2012.
4. Vinsonneau C, Launay EA, Blayau C, et al. Renal replacement therapy in adult and pediatric intensive care: Recommendations by an expert panel from the French Intensive Care Society (SRLF) with the French Society of Anesthesia Intensive Care (SFAR) French Group for Pediatric Intensive Care Emergencies (GFRUP) the French Dialysis Society (SFD). Ann Intensive Care. 2015;5(1):58.
5. Dialysis in Intensive Care Unit .Indian J Nephrol. 2012;22(7) Suppl:S43-44

CHAPTER 11

# Acute Peritoneal Dialysis in Critical Care

*Vipul Chakurkar*

## OVERVIEW

Peritoneal dialysis (PD) was first described in the 1920s for the treatment of uremia. It lost popularity owing to widespread availability of blood-based therapies. Nevertheless, PD still plays a role in treatment of critically ill acute kidney injury (AKI) patients, especially in resource-limited settings. The 0by25 initiative by Kidney Disease Improving Global Outcomes (KDIGO) focuses on preventing deaths from AKI and PD is being considered as an optimum form of renal support therapy.[1]

## COMPARISON OF ACUTE PERITONEAL DIALYSIS WITH BLOOD-BASED THERAPIES

Advantages of PD over blood-based therapies include—low cost, lesser infrastructure, and easy technique. Possibly the greatest advantage of PD over hemodialysis is hemodynamic tolerance as it is a slow and nearly continuous modality of dialysis with slow ultrafiltration that does not involve any extracorporeal circuit.

These theoretical advantages have been compared in clinical studies. Many observational studies report similar mortalities with PD and blood-based therapies. Four randomized trials compared PD with blood-based therapies (Table 1).

All these studies were done in the developing world and have their limitations. Despite these limitations,[6] overall evidence is robust enough for the International Society for Peritoneal Dialysis (ISPD) guideline:[7]

*"Peritoneal dialysis should be considered as a suitable method of continuous renal replacement therapy in patients with acute kidney injury (1B)."*

The role of PD in critical care in the current era is hard to delineate owing to multitude of issues. Nevertheless, PD can be a suitable option for many patients (Table 2).

## ACCESS TO PERITONEUM

Essential to PD is the access to peritoneal cavity. Three types of catheters can be used for PD:

1. *Flexible (Tenckhoff type) catheters*: These are large bore flexible catheters made up of polyurethane or silicon rubber. They allow better flow owing to large bore and the side holes.

**Table 1:** Randomized trials comparing PD with blood-based therapies

| *Study* | *Arogundade et al.*[2] | *Gabriel et al.*[3] | *Phu et al.*[4] | *George et al.*[5] |
|---|---|---|---|---|
| *Country* | Nigeria | Brazil | Vietnam | India |
| *Number of patients* | 40, 8 AKI,<br>Randomized to PD (4) or HD (4) | 120,<br>Randomized to HVPD (60) or daily HD (60) | 70,<br>Randomized to CVVH (34) or PD (36) | 55, Randomized to either CVVHD (29) or PD (26) |
| *Characteristics of patients* | AKI + CKD | AKI (due to ATN) | AKI due to sepsis or falciparum malaria | AKI with multi-organ involvement |
| *Sepsis* | 17% | About 45% | Yes | Yes |
| *APACHE II* | No data | 24–26 | No data | 18–19 |
| *Cause of AKI* | Mixed | Sepsis, heart failure, postoperative | Sepsis | Mixed |
| *Comparing modality* | HD | Daily HD | CVVH | CVVHD |
| *Primary outcome* | Correction of metabolic abnormalities (Not different in AKI) | Mortality<br>Renal recovery (Not different) | Correction of metabolic abnormalities (not different) | Correction of uremia (not different) |
| *Mortality* | Not different | Not different | Higher in PD (47% vs 15%) | No difference |
| *Limitations* | Low number of AKI | Flaws in randomization | PD not optimum, more peritonitis, underpowered | Small sample size |

(AKI: acute kidney injury; APACHE: acute physiology, age, and chronic health evaluation score; ATN: acute tubular necrosis; CKD: chronic kidney disease; CVVH: continuous venovenous hemofiltration; CVVHD: continuous venovenous hemodialysis; HD: hemodialysis; HVPD: high volume peritoneal dialysis; PD: peritoneal dialysis)

**Table 2:** Current role of PD in critical care

| *PD is suitable for* | *PD is unsuitable for* |
|---|---|
| Neonates and small children | Recent abdominal surgery or trauma |
| Hemodynamically unstable patients | Abdominal wall cellulitis |
| High risk of bleeding | Peritonitis |
| Liver failure | Life-threatening indication, e.g. hyperkalemia, severe metabolic acidosis |
| Raised intracranial pressure | Pulmonary edema |
| Difficult vascular access | Hypercatabolic patients |
| Patients on CAPD | Severe COPD |

(CAPD: continuous ambulatory peritoneal dialysis; COPD: chronic obstructive pulmonary disease; PD: peritoneal dialysis)

The cuffed catheters are associated with less infection. The insertion is usually done surgically (either open or laparoscopically) but bedside percutaneous insertion (using modified Seldinger technique and peel-away sheath) is safe and feasible under local anesthesia (Fig. 1).

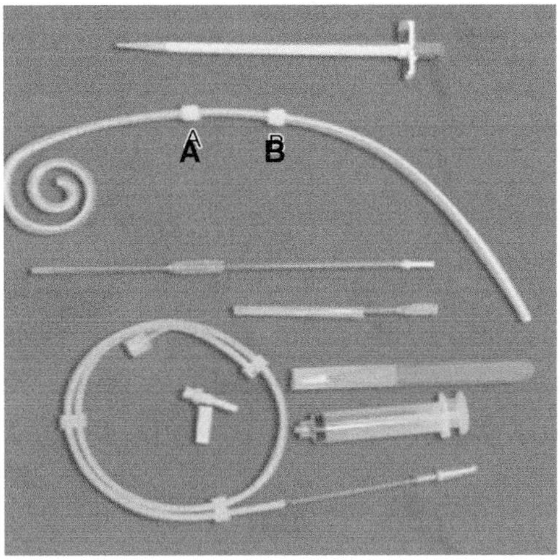


**Fig. 1:** Flexible peritoneal dialysis catheter with cuffs, coiled end, and the instruments required for percutaneous insertion of the catheter. A and B show the cuff positions.

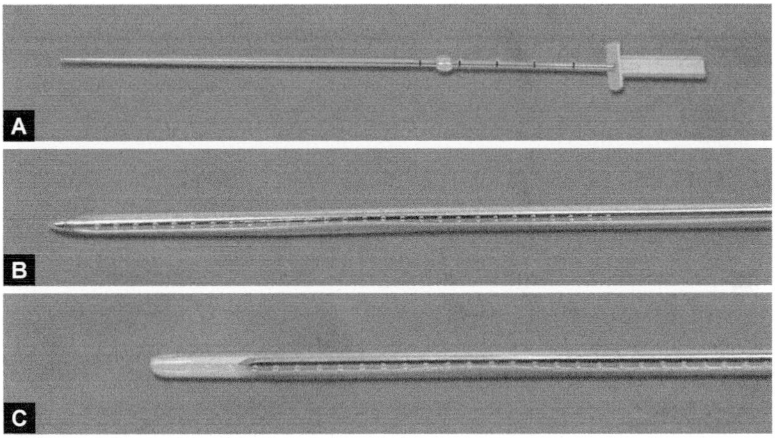


**Figs. 2A to C:** Rigid peritoneal dialysis catheter. (A) The whole catheter with a stylet; (B) Enlarged view of the intraperitoneal portion showing the "holes"; (C) When stylet is pulled back (after entry to the peritoneal cavity), the cannula is nontraumatic.

2. *Rigid catheters*: These are commonly available in India and are cost-effective. Insertion is percutaneous and involves local anesthesia, creation of artificial ascites, and insertion of the catheter with a sharp stylet to support. Though the insertion is blind, the chances of complications like bladder or intestinal puncture are very minimal, with construction of artificial ascites. Slight withdrawal of stylet into the catheter after its entry in the peritoneal cavity further minimizes the risk. The catheter is provided with side holes, all of which should be inside the peritoneal cavity to avoid fluid leak into the abdominal wall. As the catheter is not provided with a cuff and is rigid, thus it cannot be used for longer time (Figs. 2A to C).

3. *Improvised catheters*: Like nasogastric tubes, intercostal drains etc. can be inserted bedside if above two types are not available.

   *ISPD recommendation:*[7]

   *Flexible peritoneal catheters should be used for acute PD where resources and expertise exist (1C) (Optimal).*

   *It may be necessary to use rigid stylet catheters or improvised catheters in resource-poor environments where they may still be lifesaving (2D) (Minimum standard).*

## COMPONENTS OF ACUTE PERITONEAL DIALYSIS PRESCRIPTION

- Length of the dialysis session (Number of exchanges)
- Inflow, outflow, and dwell time per exchange
- Dialysate composition
- Exchange volume
- Additives
- Monitoring of fluid balance.

### "Times" in Acute Peritoneal Dialysis

- *Inflow-time*: Time required to instill fluid in the peritoneal cavity. It should be kept minimal, as no exchange is occurring during this time.
- *Outflow-time*: Time required to drain the spent dialysate from the abdominal cavity and usually takes 20–25 minutes
- *Dwell-time*: It is the time for which PD fluid stays in contact with peritoneum. The molecular exchange and ultrafiltration occur only during the dwell time. In 1-hour cycle, dwell-time is kept as 30 minutes. Shorter dwell is not efficient in removing waste products. Longer dwell increases the molecular exchange but also decreases the number of cycles that can be done. This can be compensated by increasing the volume instilled.

### Fluids for Acute Peritoneal Dialysis

The fluid promotes molecular exchange across the peritoneum. PD fluid essentially has three components: (1) water, (2) electrolytes, and (3) an osmotic agent (e.g. Dextrose). The osmotic agent determines the ultrafiltration capacity of the fluid while electrolyte concentration of the fluid tries to correct serum concentration to optimum levels.

Peritoneal dialysis fluid can be commercially available or prepared locally. ISPD guidelines[7] recommend:

*"Commercially prepared solutions should be used (1C) (Optimal). However, where resources do not permit this, locally prepared fluids may be lifesaving (2D)"*

Commercial fluids can be available in 1 L, 2 L or 5 L collapsible bags or semicollapsible bottles. They have various concentrations of dextrose, e.g. 1.5%, 1.7%, 2.5%, and 4.25% (Table 3).

Typical composition of PD fluids is described in Table 4.

**Table 3:** Osmolality and ultrafiltration capacity of various PD solutions

| *Glucose in fluid* | *Osmolality* | *UF volume per exchange over 1 hours* |
|---|---|---|
| 1.5% | 346 mOsm/L | 50–150 mL |
| 2.5% | 396 mOsm/L | 100–300 mL |
| 4.25% | 485 mOsm/L | 300–400 mL |

(UF: ultrafiltration)

**Table 4:** Composition of PD fluids

| | *Acute PD (1L) bottle* | *CAPD (2 L) bag* |
|---|---|---|
| Glucose concentration | 1.7% | 1.5, 2.5, 4.25% |
| Sodium | 130 mEq/L | 132–134 mEq/L |
| Potassium | 0 | 0–2 mEq/L |
| Chloride | 100 mEq/L | 100 mEq/L |
| Calcium | 1.5 mmol/L | 1.0–1.75 mmol/L |
| Magnesium | 0.75 mmol/L | 0.25–0.75 mmol/L |
| Bicarbonate | 35 mmol/L, as acetate | 35 mmol/L, as lactate |

(CAPD: continuous ambulatory peritoneal dialysis; PD: peritoneal dialysis)

Acute PD bottles need to be spiked each time with a Y-set while continuous ambulatory peritoneal dialysis (CAPD) bags preconnected with Y-set provide a closed circuit, thus reducing the chances of infection.

## Volume to be used

Usually 1–2 L of fluid is used. For acute PD, 1 L volume is sufficient if fluid removal is the target. As the total clearance is directly proportional to the volume exchanged per cycle, larger volume should be used if molecular exchange is the aim. Volumes larger than 2 L increase the intraperitoneal pressure thus impairing ultrafiltration in addition to causing respiratory embarrassment. Smaller adults and obese individuals tolerate smaller volumes.

## Number of Exchanges

Total number of exchanges depends on the patient requirement. Usual length is 48–72 hours with rigid acute PD catheter. The PD prescription should be rewritten every 24 hours, as patient characteristics and needs change every day. Higher chances of peritonitis are reported with treatment duration more than 60 hours.

## Additives in the Peritoneal Dialysis Fluid

- *Heparin*: It prevents fibrin clot formation. It is used when effluent is hemorrhagic or has fibrin strands and is more beneficial when added prophylactically. It poses no risk of systemic anticoagulation. Usual dose of 500 units/L is used.

- *Intraperitoneal insulin*: Used in diabetic patients on PD for glycemic control:
  - 4–5 units/L for 1.5 g/dL PD fluid
  - 5–7 units/L for 2.5 g/dL PD fluid
  - 7–10 units/L for 4.25 g/dL PD fluid.
- *Potassium*: As PD fluids are typically devoid of potassium, after 12–24 hours, hypokalemia is common. So, usually 3–4 mEq/L (2 mL/L) is added to maintain normokalemia, once serum K is <4mEq/L.

As all additives carry the risk of contamination, their use should be minimized.

## Monitoring

Though PD is a slow and continuous process, it is not without the risk. So, monitoring is essential. Fluid balance is to be monitored with strict I/O monitoring and the PD balance (in volume - out volume). Electrolytes, bicarbonate, glucose, and renal function tests (RFTs) should be monitored at least daily, if not more frequently.

## WRITING A PERITONEAL DIALYSIS PRESCRIPTION

One size does not fit all. So, PD prescription must consider the patient needs. The aims of PD treatment can be fluid removal, electrolyte correction or uremic toxin removal.

- *Correction of hyperkalemia or metabolic acidosis*: Short dwell times (30 minutes) with 1–2 L volume are essential. Peripheral bicarbonate infusion, if started, can continue till PD takes over. But frequent monitoring 4–6 hourly is needed. If no correction is obtained or the condition becomes life-threatening, blood-based therapies should be switched to.
- *Correction of uremia*: Small molecules like urea and creatinine are best cleared when dwell is kept longer (about 2–3 hours). So, a standard "CAPD-like" exchange (10–20 minutes in time, 3 hours dwell of 2L and 20–30 minutes of out-time) is used.
- *Ultrafiltration*: As glucose, the osmotic agent, is absorbed from the fluid across the peritoneum, the concentration in the peritoneum drops as the dwell-time increases, thus dropping the osmotic gradient for ultrafiltration. So, ultrafiltration is highest in the first hour and drops to zero or minus after 3–4 hours. Thus, short dwell-times with 1–2 L volume (not more than 2 L) are used for ultrafiltration. This needs patient's blood sugar to be well controlled. If the standard glucose concentrate is unable to obtain the ultrafiltration, then one can increase the ultrafiltration capacity by adding dextrose to the solution. For example, addition of 10 mL 50% dextrose solution to 1.7% 1 L bottle increases its ultrafiltration capacity by almost 100 mL/hr. But, life-threatening pulmonary edema is best treated with hemodialysis rather than with PD.

## HOW TO MEASURE DOSE?

Molecular exchange depends on two factors: (1) time of contact between PD fluid and blood and (2) the volume of PD fluid (along with membrane characteristics). The dose of PD, thus is dependent on volume of PD fluid spent over a time and is calculated as:

Dose of PD (Kt/V) = Dialysate urea × Dialysate volume/(Plasma urea × TBW)

$= D/P_{urea} \times V/TBW$

*ISPD guidelines recommend weekly Kt/V of 3.5, i.e. 0.5 daily (Optimum) with a minimum value of 0.3 per day.*[7]

## COMPLICATIONS OF PERITONEAL DIALYSIS

### Procedural Complications

- *Perforation of viscous (bladder or intestine)*: It can be prevented by making sure that bladder is empty and by creation of ascites while using rigid catheters.
- *Infusion of fluid in parietal wall*: It can be avoided by using surgical insertion of the catheter. In case rigid catheter is used, one should make sure that all the eyes of the catheter are placed inside the peritoneal cavity.
- *Bleeding*: It can occur in coagulopathic patients.

### Mechanical

- Splinting of the diaphragm and respiratory compromise
- Pleural effusion (Rt > Lt)
- Increase in hernia sac.

### Infectious

*Peritonitis* occurs in 10–40% of the patients and chances increase with duration of the PD. So, it is not advisable to continue acute PD with rigid catheters beyond 60–72 hours. Flexible catheters with 2 cuffs minimize the infection.

### Metabolic

- Hyperglycemia
- Protein loss (if more than 14 days)
- Hypokalemia (so need to monitor and add $K^+$ to the PD fluid).

Common situations, their possible causes, and the actions are described in Table 5.

## MODIFICATIONS OF PERITONEAL DIALYSIS

- *Tidal PD*: Only a part of initial dwell volume is exchanged, leaving some amount of fluid always in the peritoneal cavity thus using even the "out & in" times for exchange. This increases the clearance.
- *High volume PD*: Uses automated cycler with a flexible catheter exchanging 36–44 L of PD fluid per day.
- *Continuous flow PD*: Requires two catheters or a double lumen catheter in the abdominal cavity. Fluid is continuously exchanged at high rate increasing the clearance.

**Table 5:** Complications of peritoneal dialysis (PD).

| *Problem* | *Possible reason(s)* | *Action* |
|---|---|---|
| Poor drainage | *With poor inflow*: Mechanical problem, e.g. kink<br>*With good inflow*:<br>• Blockage by fibrin or blood clot<br>• Catheter migration<br>• Omental wrap | Removing the catheter and insertion of a new rigid catheter<br>Repositioning of the catheter either same site or different site<br>In case of omental wrap of a flexible catheter, laparoscopic or open omentectomy is needed |
| Poor drain-volume (but good flow) | • Dehydrated patient<br>• Loss of osmotic gradient | • Careful monitoring and hydration of the patient<br>• Decreasing the dwell-time or increasing the glucose concentration |
| Pericatheter leak | All the holes are not intraperitoneal | • Repositioning the catheter<br>• Purse-string suture<br>• Using the low fill-volume |
| Pain during in-flow | • Cold fluid<br>• Excessive fill volume<br>• Peritonitis | • Warming the fluid to body temperature<br>• Low fill volumes or tidal PD |
| Blood stained effluent | Minor trauma to peritoneum during insertion | • Add heparin to dialysate<br>• Usually settles with subsequent cycles |
| Fibrin in the effluent | | • Add heparin to dialysate<br>• Usually settles with subsequent cycles |
| Sensation of passing urine at the time of inflow | Bladder perforation | Remove the catheter. Drain bladder with Foley's catheter. Take surgical opinion |
| Watery diarrhea or fecal matter in the effluent | Bowel perforation | Remove the catheter<br>• Antibiotics<br>• Surgical opinion |
| Peritonitis | Improper handling of the catheter | Send PD cell count, Gram stain, culture<br>Broad spectrum antibiotics, intraperitoneal (IP), to cover both Gram positive and negative organisms.<br>Remove PD catheter if patient is unstable and septic or PD cell count not improving. Rigid catheter should be promptly removed after instillation of IP antibiotics |

## CONCLUSION

Though PD is generally considered a slow and less effective therapy, evidence, in contrary, suggests that PD is equally effective in correction of metabolic derangements and has equal mortality. With the definite niche, PD can be an alternative to blood-based therapies, especially in resource-limited settings.

## REFERENCES

1. Kher V, Srisawat N, Noiri E, et al. Prevention and therapy of acute kidney injury in the developing world. Kidney Int Rep. 2017;2(4):544-58.
2. Arogundade FA, Ishola DA Jr, Sanusi AA, et al. An analysis of the effectiveness and benefits of peritoneal dialysis and haemodialysis using Nigerian made PD fluids. Afr J Med Med Sci. 2005;34(3):227-33.

3. Gabriel DP, Caramori JT, Martim LC, et al. High volume peritoneal dialysis vs daily hemodialysis: A randomized, controlled trial in patients with acute kidney injury. Kidney Int Suppl. 2008;(108):S87-93.
4. Phu NH, Hien TT, Mai NTH, et al. Hemofiltration and peritoneal dialysis in infection-associated acute renal failure in Vietnam. N Engl J Med. 2002;347:895-902.
5. George J, Varma S, Kumar S, et al. Comparing continuous venovenous hemodiafiltration and peritoneal dialysis in critically ill patients with acute kidney injury: a pilot study. Perit Dial Int. 2011;31:422-9.
6. Chionh CY, Soni SS, Finkelstein FO, et al. Use of peritoneal dialysis in AKI: A systematic review. Clin J Am Soc Nephrol. 2013;8(10):1649-60.
7. Cullis B, Abdelraheem M, Abrahams G. et al. Peritoneal dialysis for acute kidney injury. Perit Dial Int. 2014;34(5):494-517.

## FURTHER READING

1. Ansari N. Peritoneal dialysis in renal replacement therapy for patients with acute kidney injury. Inter J Nephrol. 2011.
2. Ponce D, Balbi A, Cullis B. Acute PD: Evidence, Guidelines and Controversies. Seminar Nephrol. 2017;37(1):103-12.
3. Ponce D, Balbi AL, Finkelstein FO. Peritoneal dialysis for the treatment of acute kidney injury. In: Daugirdas JT, Blake PG, Ing TS (Eds). Handbook of Dialysis, 5th edition. US: Wolters Kluwer Health; 2015.

CHAPTER 12

# Complications and Monitoring of Renal Replacement Therapy in Acute Kidney Injury

Rajeev A Annigeri

## INTRODUCTION

Acute kidney injury (AKI) is common in intensive care unit (ICU) and is seen in 30–50% of patients. Approximately 20% of AKI patients in ICU require renal replacement therapy (RRT). The modalities of RRT commonly used in ICU are continuous renal replacement therapy (CRRT) and intermittent hemodialysis (IHD). Peritoneal dialysis is infrequently used in ICU in adults. CRRT is generally reserved for patients with severe hemodynamic instability. Sustained low efficiency dialysis (SLED) as a hybrid therapy has evolved recently and is being used increasingly in patients with mild hemodynamic instability. However, there is a wide variation in the practice of RRT in ICUs across the world, which is influenced by type of patient populations, cost and the availability of technology, expertise, and resources. Though CRRT has several practical and clinical advantages over IHD or SLED, none of the randomized studies have shown a significant survival benefit with CRRT. In the light of such results, some have raised the concern that the complications arising from the use of CRRT may negate its potential benefits.[1]

Dialysis therapy removes solutes of certain size which are permeable through the pores of the membrane and adds specified solutes to maintain the physiological composition of the plasma. The RRT in AKI is associated with several complications and hence should not be considered as innocuous therapy. A comprehensive knowledge of the potential complications associated with RRT would enable the clinician to prevent them or treat them early, to minimize their harm. The monitoring of RRT serves several purposes such as—(1) the proper application of the prescribed therapy, (2) the targets of therapy are achieved, and (3) complications are either prevented or treated early to minimize their adverse effects.

## COMPLICATIONS OF RENAL REPLACEMENT THERAPY

The complications related to RRT can be classified based on the source and their nature, as shown in Table 1.

### Complications Related to Vascular Access

The vascular access commonly used for RRT in ICU in order of preference is jugular vein followed by femoral vein. The subclavian vein is not preferred in view of increased risk of central vein

**Table 1:** Complications associated with renal replacement therapy in acute kidney injury.

| *Source of complication* | *Nature of complication* |
|---|---|
| Vascular access | Bleeding and hematoma<br>Arteriovenous fistula, aneurism<br>Pneumothorax<br>Venous thrombosis<br>Bloodstream infection |
| Dialysis circuit | Clotting of the filter and tubing, with blood loss<br>Hypothermia<br>Immune activation<br>Endotoxemia |
| Dialysis therapy | Electrolyte disturbances: Hypokalemia, hyper or hyponatremia, hypocalcemia, hypophosphatemia<br>Acid–base disturbances<br>Removal of drugs<br>Loss of protein and micronutrients |
| Anticoagulation | Bleeding<br>Heparin-induced thrombocytopenia<br>Metabolic disturbances related to RCA |
| Physiology of patient | Hypotension<br>Cardiac arrhythmias<br>Increased intracranial tension<br>Delayed renal recovery |
| Operator and the machine | Prescription errors<br>Errors in compounding solutions<br>Administration errors<br>Errors in fluid balance |

(RCA: regional citrate anticoagulation)

stenosis. The serious complications of vascular access are pneumothorax, arterial puncture causing arteriovenous fistula and aneurism and bleeding which may lead to hematoma, hemothorax, and blood loss. The prolonged use of femoral catheters may result in venous thrombosis and pulmonary embolism. The ultrasound guidance to insert dialysis catheter reduces the risk of complications and hence should be used when available. However, the most common complication of vascular access is the catheter-related bloodstream infections (CRBSI). The prolonged length of catheter use and femoral site, especially in obese patients, increases the risk of CRBSI. The dialysis catheter removal should be considered when dialysis is no longer needed and for temporary jugular catheter after 3 weeks and femoral catheter after 5 days. The incidence of CRBSI is 2.5 times higher in AKI patients receiving RRT compared to non-AKI patients in ICU.[2] A new episode of CRBSI in ICU increases the risk of death by 12–25% and increases the duration and cost of hospitalization significantly.

## Complications Related to Dialysis Circuit

The extracorporeal circuit of CRRT and IHD consist of tubings and dialysis filter. The blood exposed to extracorporeal circuit triggers clotting cascade and the common sites of clotting of circuit are dialysis filter and venous drip chamber. The clotting of the circuit results in loss of blood, which could be substantial, if circuit clots frequently. Hypothermia is a problem in CRRT if the dialysis fluids are not warmed by an external warmer which may not be available in some CRRT machines and occurs in ~30–65% of patients. Severe hypothermia can cause coagulopathy and altered drug pharmacodynamics. Hypothermia can be prevented or minimized by external warming of the body and warming the dialysis fluids by an external warmer in CRRT. The exposure of blood to the extracorporeal circuit induces an immune response resulting in inflammatory state. The short-term impact of such an inflammatory activation in critically ill patients is not clear. On a rare occasion, an acute allergic reaction can occur after initiation of dialysis, more so with bioincompatible membranes. The angiotensin-converting enzyme (ACE) inhibitors should be avoided in patients when AN-69 dialysis membrane is used for RRT, which can induce an anaphylactic reaction. The quality of dialysis fluid is important in IHD. The contamination of dialysis fluid with endotoxin may result in back diffusion of endotoxin from dialysate fluids into blood circulation when high flux dialysis is used. In case online hemodiafiltration is used in ICU, ultrapure quality of the dialysis water should be maintained at all times.

## Complications Related to Dialysis Therapy

The dialysis process can remove several essential solutes and their deficiency can occur if these are not adequately replenished.

### *Electrolyte Disturbances*

The electrolyte and divalent ion disturbances are frequent in RRT, though severe complications are rare. They are more frequent when custom-made fluids are used in CRRT, compared to the use of commercially available fluids, wherein the wrong choice of fluids and human errors in compounding the dialysis fluids can occur. Hypophosphatemia and hypomagnesemia are the two most common electrolyte abnormalities to occur in CRRT, which can be prevented by dialysis fluids with phosphate and magnesium that are available recently. The incidences of electrolyte disturbances in major reported studies are shown in Table 2.

**Table 2:** Incidence of new onset adverse events during continuous renal replacement therapy (CRRT).

| | *Akhoundi et al.*[3,a] | *VA/ATN study*[5,b] | *RENAL study*[4,a] | *Gaudry et al.*[6,b] | *ELAIN study*[7,c] |
|---|---|---|---|---|---|
| Hypokalemia | 4% | 6% | 24.1% | 22% | - |
| Hyperkalemia | 7% | 3.8% | - | 5.5% | - |
| Hyponatremia | 0.6% | 5.2% | - | - | - |
| Hypernatremia | 3% | 0.8% | - | - | - |
| Hypophosphatemia | 34% | 14.2% | 59.5% | 18.6% | - |
| Hypocalcemia | 22% | 10% | - | - | 63.2% |
| Hypercalcemia | 23% | 2.1% | - | - | - |
| Metabolic acidosis | - | 6%% | - | - | - |
| Metabolic alkalosis | - | 3.5% | - | - | - |

(a: CRRT; b: mixed CRRT and IRRT; c: CRRT with citrate anticoagulation)

### *Acid–base Disturbances*

Lactic acidosis is the most common type of metabolic acidosis in patients receiving RRT and other types are seen less frequently. The dialysis fluids containing lactate may be avoided in patients with significant lactic acidosis, poor muscle mass, and liver failure. The lack of conversion of lactate to bicarbonate in them may result in accumulation of $H^+$, thereby worsening acidosis. The dialysate bicarbonate concentration has an impact on the correction of acidosis. In hemofiltration, bicarbonate concentration should be more than that of plasma to correct acidosis, since sieving coefficient of bicarbonate is more than 1.

### *Nutritional Losses*

Significant amount of amino acids and proteins are lost during RRT, which may contribute to the negative nitrogen balance in them. The degree of loss of protein is influenced by pore size of the filter, convective dialysis, intensity and duration of RRT, and degree of catabolism associated with critical illness. The glucose-free dialysis fluids can infrequently cause hypoglycemia due to loss of glucose and induce gluconeogenesis which uses amino acid as the substrate. Several water-soluble vitamins and minerals and micronutrients are lost during RRT and it is essential to supplement them, especially in whom RRT is needed for prolonged period.

### *Removal of Drugs*

The altered pharmacokinetics of drugs due to the removal of drugs during RRT has received much attention recently. Adequate dose delivery of drugs, especially that of antibiotics in septic patients is critical for recovery from illness, as well as prevention of emergence of drug-resistant bacteria. Vasopressor clearance also can be substantial, especially when the vasopressors are delivered close to the dialysis catheter. The drug level monitoring should be done when available, especially in very sick patients. However, such a provision is scarce even in developed countries. Recent evidence indicates that the dose of antibiotics prescribed in CRRT based on the standard recommendation guidelines is likely to miss the dosing target by a wide margin and often results in under-dosing. Hence it is better to prescribe higher doses than recommended at least during the first 48 hours during CRRT to prevent under-dosing in critically ill patients.

## Complications Related to Patient's Physiology

### *Hypotension*

Hypotension is one of the most common adverse events occurring during RRT. Hypotension can precipitate an acute coronary event or cerebrovascular accident in a susceptible patient. Also, it can cause gut ischemia, leading to Gram-negative sepsis and may delay the recovery from AKI. Sometimes it is difficult to differentiate between hypotension induced by RRT and that due to comorbidity and critical illness. Moreover, there is no clear established definition of hypotension related to RRT in critically ill patients, which is the reason for a wide variability in reported incidence of RRT related hypotension in ICU. Akhoundi et al. defined hypotension while on CRRT, as a mean arterial pressure (MAP) <60 mm Hg or a systolic blood pressure <90 mm Hg or need for intervention such as intravenous fluid boluses or increase in inotrope dose to counter the fall in blood pressure. In their study, hypotension occurred in 43% of patients within one hour of initiation of RRT.[3] Compared to IHD, hypotension occurs less frequently in CRRT, though patients with most hemodynamic instability are chosen for CRRT. In general, the incidence of hypotension in CRRT is 50%, 30–70% in IHD, and 40–60% in SLED. Several factors contribute to the development of hypotension during RRT, such as rapid fluid removal that is not compensated by vascular refilling, higher intensity of dialysis, poor vasoconstriction, hypoalbuminemia, hyponatremic dialysis fluids, acetate dialysate, and cardiac stunning. Contrary to the common belief, the higher blood flow rates do not contribute to the causation of hypotension during RRT.

### *Cardiac Arrhythmias*

Cardiac arrhythmias are also common and a large randomized study comparing low intensity and high intensity CRRT in AKI reported 34.7% incidence of arrhythmias during CRRT, which required treatment and 26% incidence of arrhythmias causing hemodynamic instability.[4]

### *Renal Recovery*

Transient or overt hypotension during RRT may compromise the renal perfusion and may result in repeated ischemic insults to the kidney. Kidney biopsies in patients with poor recovery from AKI showed areas of new acute tubular injury indicating a possible role of RRT in delayed recovery from AKI. The modalities of RRT causing least hemodynamic disturbance such as CRRT and peritoneal dialysis have shown better renal recovery and less dialysis dependency in AKI.

### *Complications due to Anticoagulation*

Heparin is commonly used for systemic anticoagulation in RRT and is associated with increased risk of bleeding in critically ill. Regional citrate anticoagulation (RCA) for CRRT is commonly used in developed countries. The RCA reduces the risk of bleeding and the need for transfusions. Anticoagulation free RRT is least associated with risk of bleeding, but reduces the lifespan of the filter as well as the dialysis efficacy over time. The RCA is complex and is associated with medication errors, when custom-made solutions are used. In addition, metabolic complications such as hypocalcemia, metabolic acidosis as well as alkalosis are not uncommon when RCA is used for CRRT.

## Complications Related to Operator and Machine

Several complications due to human errors in prescribing, compounding the solutions, and administration can occur during RRT. In addition, malfunction of the dialysis machine and mishandling of alarms from the machine may potentially cause harm to the patient.

The errors in compounding the solutions can occur commonly, when custom-made solutions are for CRRT and can have deleterious effects on patients, including rare fatalities.[8] The use of pre-printed CRRT sets, calculation safety checks, and standardized practices may reduce the incidence as well as severity of CRRT-related medical errors. The use of commercially prepared solutions has markedly reduced the medication errors in CRRT. However, many commercially available CRRT solutions do not contain potassium, magnesium, and phosphate and they need to be supplemented. Errors in compounding these supplements can lead to electrolyte abnormalities. Though the safety and reliability of CRRT machines have greatly improved in recent years, there still remains a potential for fluid balance errors during CRRT. The alarms from the machines with regard to fluid balance errors should not be ignored and over riding the alarms can result in harm.

## MONITORING OF RENAL REPLACEMENT THERAPY

The monitoring of RRT is an essential component of therapy to ensure adequate and safe delivery of therapy. It also helps to modify therapy to the changing physiological demands, metabolic needs, and the intrinsic capacity of the kidneys in an individual patient.

The physiological and biochemical derangements may be categorized into critical, moderate, and mild or no derangements based on the principles suggested by Common Terminology Criteria for Adverse Events (CTCAE) proposed by National Institute of Health[9] and are illustrated in Figure 1.

### Components of Monitoring of Therapy

Monitoring of therapy broadly involves two categories: (1) Monitoring patient-related physiological and biochemical parameters and (2) Monitoring the performance and safety concerns of the extracorporeal circuit. They encompass several components and are shown in Box 1.

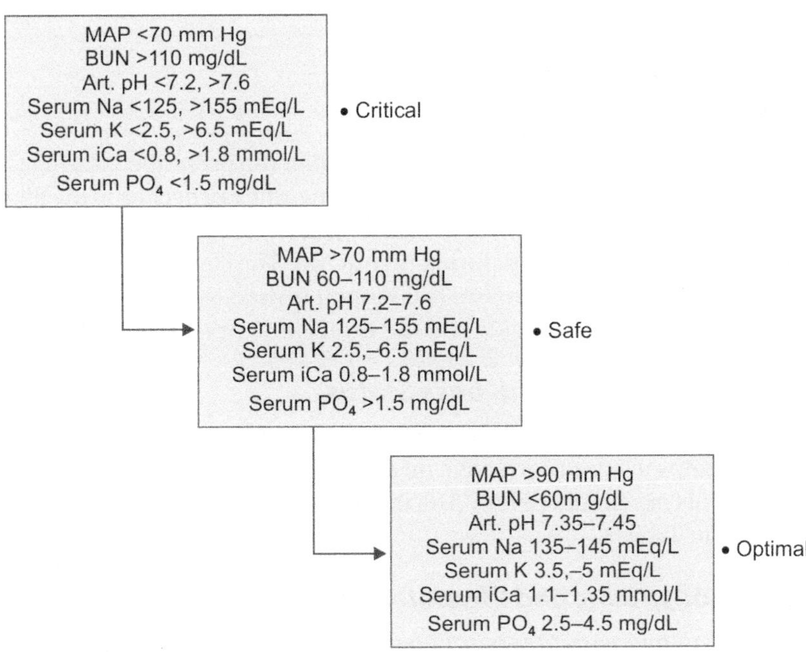


**Fig. 1:** Categorization of degree of physiological derangements in AKI while on RRT.

(AKI: acute kidney injury; BUN: blood urea nitrogen; MAP: mean arterial pressure; RRT: renal replacement therapy)

**Box 1:** Components of monitoring suggested for monitoring in acute kidney injury patients receiving renal replacement therapy.

*Monitoring patient-related factors*
- Hemodynamic parameters:
  - Blood pressure
  - Heart rate
  - Cardiac function
- Physiologic status:
  - Respiratory function
  - Urine output
  - Intracranial pressure
  - Coagulation parameters
  - Liver function
  - Organ failure score
- Solute clearance
- Blood concentration of electrolyte and divalent ions
- Serum sodium, potassium, calcium, phosphorus and magnesium
- Acid–base status
- Fluid balance and organ edema
- Body temperature

*Monitoring extracorporeal circuit*
- Vascular access performance
- Filter performance
- Monitoring circuit pressures
- Safety alarms of machine
- Monitoring "down time" in continuous renal replacement therapy (CRRT)
- Anticoagulation effect

## *Monitoring Solute Clearance*

The delivered dose of solute clearance is often lower than the prescribed during CRRT, due to "down time" effect and reduced solute clearance over time, due to a decline in the filter efficiency. The periodic measurement of small solute clearance such as urea is essential to ensure that the prescribed dose of dialysis is delivered during RRT in AKI. The clearance of urea is used for the dose delivery and blood side urea kinetics (Kt/V urea) is used to measure the delivered dose in IHD and SLED, whereas dialysate side kinetics is recommended for CRRT (KD, mL/min).

## *Monitoring Electrolyte and Acid–base Status*

The electrolyte and acid-base disturbances are common while on RRT and hence need close monitoring, which helps to adapt corrective measures to prevent harmful adverse events. The proposed frequency of tests should be based on the need of the individual patients and proposed frequency is shown in Table 3.

## *Monitoring Hemodynamic and Physiological Status of the Patient*

Monitoring hemodynamic parameters such as blood pressure, heart rate, cardiac rhythm, and body temperature constitute standard monitoring during RRT. Continuous monitoring of blood pressure is done when arterial line is in place. Automated blood pressure monitoring

**Table 3:** Proposed intensity of biochemical monitoring during renal replacement therapy based on the grade of derangements.

| | *Grade 3*[a] | *Grade 2*[b] | *Grade 1*[c] |
|---|---|---|---|
| Blood urea nitrogen | Once daily | Once daily | Once in 2 days |
| Serum creatinine | Once daily | Once daily | Once 2 days |
| Serum potassium | Q4–6 hours | Q8–24 hours | Once daily |
| Serum sodium | Q6–12 hours | Once daily | Q24–48 hours |
| Serum calcium or ionized calcium | Q6 hourly | Q6–8 hours | Q48–72 hours |
| Serum phosphorus | Q24 hours | Q24–48 hours | Q72 hours or less |
| ABG or VBG analysis | Q4–6 hours | Q8–24 hours | Once daily |

(a: critical derangements; b: moderate derangements; c: mild or no derangements; ABG: arterial blood gas; VBG: venous blood gas)

has largely replaced manual measurement of blood pressure in ICU, done at frequent intervals of 5–15 minutes. However, blood pressure measures by automated machine may be erroneous and hence they should be periodically verified by manual measurements. More sophisticated hemodynamic measures, such as cardiac output monitors, pulmonary artery catheterization, are not generally required. Measures such as central venous pressure, bioimpedance analysis, blood volume monitor during RRT, and atrial natriuretic peptide are used to guide fluid removal, but currently their clinical utility is uncertain.

The physiologic state of the critically ill patients has a significant impact on their outcome. Quantification of acute physiologic derangements is assessed by several clinical scores, which have been validated in critically ill patients. Serial measures of acute illness scores provide valuable information regarding changing demands of the patients. In the absence of superiority of over other score, a scoring system which is easy to perform may be adapted for clinical use. A study showed that a rise in the Sequential Organ Failure Assessment (SOFA) score by 30% is associated with mortality of >50%. The renal capacity is generally measured by the amount of urine and would help clinician to guide to consider stopping RRT. A spontaneous urine output of >400 mL/day or diuretic aided urine output of >2,300 mL/day are useful markers to consider a trial of withdrawal from RRT.

## Monitoring Fluid Balance

Fluid overload is common in critically ill patients and in AKI and is associated with increased rate of complications and mortality in ICU. Fluid overload can be expressed as percentage and is calculated by the formula:

*Percent fluid overload = (Total fluid in – Total fluid out)/admission weight × 100*

The significance of fluid balance is illustrated by the fact that fluid accumulation of more than 10% of body weight and prolonged duration of fluid accumulation is associated with increased mortality in ICU.[10] Monitoring the cumulative balance of fluids would help to achieve fluid balance close to neutral on RRT, which may improve outcomes. CRRT appears to be more efficient in achieving better fluid balance than IHD; however, SLED appears to be equivalent

**Table 4:** Pressure monitors in the circuit of continuous renal replacement therapy and the causes and consequences of pressures exceeding the limits.

| *Pressure* | *Normal* | *Limit* | *Causes to exceed limit* | *Consequences if exceeds limit* |
|---|---|---|---|---|
| Access | −30 to −150 | −250 | Poor flow though catheter, increased blood pump speed | Vein wall injury, hemolysis |
| Filter | +80 to +400 | +500 | Increased resistance to post blood pump flow, increased blood flow rates | Risk of pushing clot forward/ circuit blood leaks |
| Effluent | +50 to −150 | | – | – |
| TMP | 0 to +200 | +300 | High UF rates, clogged membrane pores, use of low flux filter, high blood compartment pressure | Membrane rupture, blood in effluent |
| Return | +50 to +250 | +350 | Increased resistance to post blood pump flow, increased blood flow rates | Risk of pushing clot forward/ circuit blood leaks |

(TMP: transmembrane pressure; UF: ultrafiltration) (All pressures expressed as mm Hg)

to CRRT in this respect.[11] Several methods are used to guide the fluid removal in AKI patients. Use of chest radiography, natriuretic peptides, bioimpedance analysis, thoracic ultrasound, and vena cava measurements by ultrasound have been proposed as a guide to prescribe fluid removal during RRT, but they have not been rigorously studied for routine clinical application.

### *Monitoring Extracorporeal Circuit*

The monitoring of extracorporeal circuit is essential to maintain adequate flow through the circuit, which is critical for adequate and safe delivery of RRT. The monitoring involves function of vascular access, filter, safety alarms, and pressure measurements at various points in the circuit. The various circuit pressure measures in CRRT, their limits and the causes, and the consequences of exceeding the limits are shown in Table 4. The filter clotting is common when TMP exceeds 200 mm Hg and hence when this is reached the filter may be changed routinely. The dialysis efficiency should be tested when TMP is close to 200 mm Hg and if dialysate/plasma (D/P) urea is <0.8, the filter may be changed to reduce the risk of under-dialysis.

### *Anticoagulation*

The monitoring of anticoagulation is dealt elsewhere.

## CONCLUSION

Complications related to RRT in AKI are common, which may sometimes mitigate the enormous benefits provided by RRT. The prevention of therapy-related complications should be one of the principal goals of RRT. The monitoring of RRT facilitates the effective delivery of therapy, as well as prevention and early correction of complications due to RRT.

## REFERENCES

1. Finkel KW, Podoll AS. Complications of continuous renal replacement therapy. Semin Dial. 2009;22(2): 155-9.

2. Hoste EA, Blot SI, Lameire NH, et al. Effect of nosocomial bloodstream infection on the outcome of critically ill patients with acute renal failure treated with renal replacement therapy. J Am Soc Nephrol. 2004;15:454-62.
3. Akhoundi A, Singh B, Vela M, et al. Incidence of adverse events during continuous renal replacement therapy. Blood Purif. 2015;39(4):333-9.
4. RENAL Replacement Therapy Study Investigators; Bellomo R, Cass A, Cole L, et al. Intensity of continuous renal-replacement therapy in critically ill patients. N Engl J Med. 2009;361(17):1627-38.
5. VA/NIH Acute Renal Failure Trial Network; Palevsky PM, Zhang JH, O'Connor TZ, et al. Intensity of renal support in critically ill patients with acute kidney injury. N Engl J Med. 2008;359(1):7-20.
6. Gaudry S, Hajage D, Schortgen F, et al. AKIKI Study Group. Initiation strategies for renal-replacement therapy in the intensive care unit. N Engl J Med. 2016;375(2):122-33.
7. Zarbock A, Kellum JA, Schmidt C, et al. Effect of Early vs Delayed Initiation of Renal Replacement Therapy on Mortality in Critically Ill Patients With Acute Kidney Injury: The ELAIN Randomized Clinical Trial. JAMA. 2016;315(20):2190-9.
8. Barletta JF, Barletta GM, Brophy PD, et al. Medication errors and patient complications with continuous renal replacement therapy. Pediatr Nephrol. 2006;21(6):842-5.
9. US Department of Health and Human Services, National Institutes of Health, National Cancer Institute. (2009). Common Terminology Criteria for Adverse Events (CTCAE) Version 4.0. Available from https://www.acrin.org/Portals/0/Administration/Regulatory/CTCAE_4.02_2009-09-15_QuickReference_5x7.pdf [Last Accessed June 2019].
10. Bouchard J, Soroko SB, Chertow GM, et al. Program to Improve Care in Acute Renal Disease (PICARD) Study Group. Fluid accumulation, survival and recovery of kidney function in critically ill patients with acute kidney injury. Kidney Int. 2009;76(4):422-7.
11. Zhang L, Yang J, Eastwood GM, et al. Extended Daily Dialysis Versus Continuous Renal Replacement Therapy for Acute Kidney Injury: A Meta-analysis. Am J Kidney Dis. 2015;66(2):322-30.

CHAPTER 13

# Chronic Kidney Disease Patient in ICU

*Tarun K Jeloka*

## WHY IS IT IMPORTANT TO DISCUSS CHRONIC KIDNEY DISEASE IN INTENSIVE CARE UNIT FORUM?

Acute kidney injury (AKI) is regularly being discussed in critical care conferences as it is an important cause of increased morbidity in intensive cell unit (ICU) patients. There are many causes of AKI, of which, sepsis is one of the most important cause. However, there are increasing numbers of patients with pre-existing renal dysfunction [chronic kidney disease (CKD)] who get admitted with acute critical illnesses in ICU. These patients have increased risk of acute kidney function deterioration because of prerenal, renal or at times postrenal causes leading to acute on CKD. In fact, CKD is an independent and strongest risk factor (× 10 times) for acute on CKD.[1] Literature review shows 12–35% patients in ICU have acute on CKD. Apart from CKD, in a prospective analysis, it was seen that 3.4% ICU admissions were of end-stage renal disease (ESRD) patients. The demographics of these ESRD patients is different. When these ESRD patients were compared to general population getting admitted in ICU, ESRD patients were younger, twice as common to have diabetes, peripheral vascular disease, and sepsis, and are admitted for nonsurgical cause.[2]

## OUTCOMES OF CKD PATIENTS ADMITTED IN ICU

It has been seen that individuals with low estimated glomerular filtration rate (eGFR) or proteinuria (both are features of CKD) have higher risk of acute on CKD. Those having stage 3b (eGFR 30 to 45 mL/min) have 5 times and those in stage 4 (eGFR 15 to 30 mL/min), have 20 times increased risk of acute on CKD as compared to patients with eGFR >60 mL/min.[3] Further, patients with proteinuria between +2 and +4 have 7-fold increased risk of need for renal replacement therapy (RRT).[4] It is important to know about pre-existing kidney disease because the outcomes of AKI patients and those with acute on CKD are different. In a study, need for dialysis and in-hospital mortality were more common with AKI than with acute on CKD.[5] Overall hospital mortality was 10% in nonrenal, 16% in ESRD, and 40% in AKI. It also showed that ESRD was not an independent factor associated with mortality.

## WHY CKD PATIENTS ARE DIFFERENT?

It is known that CKD patients are a different population altogether and need appropriate attention over and above other ICU patients. They have higher comorbidities like diabetes, hypertension, peripheral vascular disease, and malnutrition. CKD induces structural and physiological changes in other organ systems. Because of all this, these patients are at high risk of early worsening of various organ functions, and make assessment of organ dysfunction difficult. It leads to increased morbidity and mortality. Pulmonary edema and sepsis are the most frequent causes of admissions and cardiovascular and sepsis are the two most common causes of death in CKD patients in ICU. The changes in various organ systems can be summarized as below.

### Cardiovascular System

Patients with CKD have higher incidence of left ventricular hypertrophy, coronary artery disease, pulmonary hypertension, and dilated cardiomyopathy. Interpretation of cardiac enzymes, especially in asymptomatic patients, is also difficult, as both troponins are excreted by kidneys and their levels may be high as such. Increasing levels however, have prognostic significance of structural heart disease and increased risk of major cardiac events. Similarly, brain natriuretic peptide (BNP), a marker of heart failure, also requires caution in interpretation.

### Immunological System

Chronic kidney disease leads to attenuated inflammatory and immunological response, which contributes to higher risk of infections. Antimicrobial resistance further contributes to poor outcome of these patients.

### Pulmonary System

Chronic kidney disease confers poor compliance to lungs, increases incidence of pulmonary edema and pleural effusion, and obstructive sleep apnea (as high as 60%), which makes the management in ICU challenging. Mechanical ventilation per se can also cause renal injury.

### Renal System

With pre-existing renal dysfunction, higher dose of diuretic is required for similar effect. Frusemide is more kaliuretic and hence, when required, frusemide is better than torsemide in managing hyperkalemia. Infusion has been found to have better diuresis as compared to split doses. However, infusion should not be endless and if no results, should be withdrawn. "Frusemide challenge" is predictive of progression of kidney injury. A urine output of <200 mL in 2 hours after a 1 to 1.5 mg/kg IV Frusemide, suggests poorer renal prognosis and possible progression of kidney injury. It is also associated with increased need for RRT and increased mortality.

### Gastrointestinal System

Chronic kidney disease is associated with altered gut microbiome, poor gastrointestinal (GI) motility, and increased incidence of hepatitis B and C, especially in dialysis population.

### Others

Chronic kidney disease is associated with electrolyte imbalances which makes the management more difficult. There may be disorders of sodium, potassium, calcium, magnesium, and phosphate. Early assessment and careful fluid selection may ameliorate iatrogenic complications. CKD patients also have pre-existing metabolic acidosis, which may make acid–base assessment difficult and mixed patterns may need detailed evaluation and accurate management.

## MANAGEMENT OF CKD PATIENTS IN ICU

The initial resuscitation of critically ill patient requires an intravenous (IV) access, appropriate IV fluids, hemodynamic and cardiac monitoring, and specific treatment. The most important part of management in CKD patient is to AVOID iatrogenic complications. The following care will avoid iatrogenic complications while managing a CKD patient in ICU.

### Intravenous Access

It is recommended to preserve one, preferably nondominant, arm from cannulation for future need of arteriovenous fistula (AVF). It is best to avoid peripherally inserted central catheter (PICC) lines also for the same reason. All nursing staffs and junior doctors should be sensitive in avoiding lines in both the limbs. It is better to put in central line in an expected prolonged stay of a critically ill patient who may need long parenteral antibiotics, rather than putting several peripheral lines one after the other. Triple lumen hemodialysis catheters can also be used when dialysis is expected, where third port can be used for medicines. However while on dialysis, one should be cautious in administering drugs, especially inotropes, which should not be administered through the same line as it may be sucked in extracorporeal circuit, making the patient devoid of lifesaving drugs. Use of double lumen or triple lumen catheter is on the discretion of intensivist and has similar risk of infections. If a patient has AVF, it should be marked and care should be practiced not to apply ID band or restraints, which can compress the vein and lead to thrombosis of AVF. At times, in an unstable patient, it is better to put a dialysis catheter rather than use AVF, so as to avoid infiltration/hematoma because of sudden movements during dialysis.

### Fluids

One should be careful in advising fluids for resuscitation, as many may be in positive fluid balance because of pre-existing CKD. Early goal directed therapy has to be modified and there is need for regular reassessment of fluid status. Though "Balanced" solution is better in general ICU patients, "Normal saline" may be required based on serum potassium. Starch solutions, for resuscitation, are absolutely contraindicated for higher risk of kidney injury and need for RRT. Albumin as resuscitation fluid has limited role in ICU patients. Noninvasive methods of monitoring like bioimpedance or ultrasonography and invasive hemodynamic monitoring may be helpful in management of these patients.

## Monitoring

Monitoring is an integral part of management of ICU patients. One should avoid one, preferably nondominant, arm for BP cuff as repeated frequent BP monitoring leads to swelling of the limb. Frequency of monitoring can be reduced as per need of patient. Blood gases are integral part of management of ICU patients but lead to thrombosis of radial artery, which might be required in future for AVF creation. It has been shown that venous blood gas (VBG) is good enough as compared to arterial blood gas in day to day management, except in cases of severe circulatory and respiratory failure. pH is higher in arterial blood gas (ABG) by 0.03 and $PvCO_2$ and $TCO_2$ are higher in VBG.

## Treatment

Chronic kidney disease patients are already on multiple medicines. Previous such medicines should be looked into and relevant medicines continued. Blood pressure medicines may need to be continued or modified. Diabetes medicines may need to change to insulin treatment. Other supportive medicines like phosphate binders and erythropoiesis stimulating agents may be stopped as per need. Nephrotoxic drugs including nonsteroidal anti-inflammatory drugs and antibiotics like aminoglycosides are better avoided.

Depending on eGFR, several drugs especially antibiotic dosing need to be adjusted. If the patient is, or goes on to RRT, drug dosing has to be readjusted depending on the modality of RRT. Of all the RRTs, continuous forms of RRT like venovenous hemodiafiltration (CVVHDF) can remove maximum concentration of drugs and hence the dose requirement is like of normal GFR. Midaz, e.g., including its metabolite, is not renally cleared and not even in continuous renal replacement therapy (CRRT) and hence needs reduced dosing. Fentanyl is not cleared by hemodialysis. Radiocontrast is better avoided as far as possible and other alternative form of imaging may be resorted to. If radiocontrast is necessary, one should avoid dehydration. N-acetylcysteine prophylaxis, prior to contrast, can be advised for whatsoever benefit it may have. MRI Gadolinium contrast is also contraindicated if eGFR is <30 mL/min. It may lead to life-threatening "nephrogenic systemic fibrosis".

## Specific Management

Renal replacement therapy is required in about 13.5% of patients admitted in ICU. The indications could be absolute and relative. Absolute indications include hyperkalemia, metabolic acidosis, pulmonary edema, and encephalopathy not responding to medical management. In ICU, there are more of relative indications like metabolic or fluid homeostasis. The choice of RRT can be intermittent hemodialysis, slow low efficiency dialysis, CRRT or even peritoneal dialysis (PD). None of these modalities have proved to be better to each other in terms of survival benefits. CRRT is more often a choice for hemodynamically compromised patients. PD is another good option especially in resource poor centers. PD has been shown to be equally effective in solute removal as any other forms of extracorporeal therapies. Modifications in PD, like "tidal" or "continuous flow", or "high volume" PD, have been shown to have comparable results, even to CRRTs.[6] Hence, the decision is based on availability, cost, comfort of intensivist, and other logistics.

Vascular access for dialysis can be internal jugular catheter, femoral or subclavian in that order. AVF, if present, can be used if patient is stable (not hypotensive or restless) or could be kept at rest for the risk of infiltration and hematoma with patient movements. PD catheter can be inserted percutaneously at bed side. Cuffed silicone catheter is preferred to stiff PD catheters. Renal transplant recipient, whenever gets admitted in ICU, should be referred to a nephrologist, preferably primary transplant physician, so as to continue or modify the dose of immunosuppressants.

### Nutrition

This is the most neglected part in management of CKD patients in ICU, especially in initial few days. Nutrition is an important determinant of outcome of these patients. The nutritional requirement should be individualized by a dietician in consultation with the nephrologist. As against the usual low protein diet for CKD patients, these patients in ICU are catabolic and need normal to high protein diet. Micronutrient supplements are also required. If the patient status changes, like if they go on dialysis, their requirement also changes. All forms of RRT lead to protein losses. Hemodialysis can lose 0.5–15 g/day as compared to 5–10 g/day in hemofiltration. Such losses have to be replaced to avoid protein–energy malnutrition.

## CONCLUSION

More and more number of CKD patients are getting admitted in intensive care units and they have pre-existing compromised organs. Any acute event, medical or surgical, can push these organs to clinically relevant organ dysfunction. Further, acute injury in CKD patients may leave patient dialysis dependent or may set a new and lower baseline renal function. Management of such patients needs critical evaluation and insight into their treatment. Proper training of staff can prevent iatrogenic complications in CKD patients admitted in ICU.

## REFERENCES

1. Palevsky PM, Weisbord SD. Critical care nephrology: It's not just acute kidney injury. JASN. 2009;20(11): 2281-2.
2. Strijack B, Mojica J, Sood M, et al. Outcomes of chronic dialysis patients admitted to the intensive care unit. JASN. 2009;20(11):2441-7.
3. Hsu CY, Ordonez JD, Chertow GM, et al. The risk of acute renal failure in patients with chronic kidney disease. Kidney Int. 2008;74(1):101-7.
4. Huang TM, Wu VC, Young GH, et al. Preoperative proteinuria predicts adverse renal outcomes after coronary artery bypass grafting. JASN. 2011;22(1):156-63.
5. Prakash J, Rathore SS, Arora P, et al. Comparison of clinical characteristics of acute kidney injury versus acute-on-chronic renal failure: Our experience in a developing country. Hongkong J Nephrol. 2015;17(1):14-20.
6. Ponce D, Gobo-Oliveira M, Balbi AL. Peritoneal dialysis treatment modality option in acute kidney injury. Blood Purif. 2017;43:173-8.

CHAPTER 14

# Drug Dosing on Renal Replacement Therapy

*Jignesh N Shah, Vishwanath C Patil*

## INTRODUCTION

Drugs to be efficacious need to have therapeutic plasma concentration. Critical illness significantly affects the pharmacokinetic (PK) and pharmacodynamics (PDs) of drugs. Associated organ dysfunctions particularly acute kidney injury (AKI) will also affect drug clearance. Often it is difficult to exactly predict residual renal function and extent of nonrenal/enzymatic clearances. More so, for a critically ill patient requiring hemodialysis (HD), drug dosing is multifactorial and complex. Typically, for patients on renal replacement therapy (RRT), glomerular filtration rate (GFR) is supposed to be less than 10–15 mL/min and dose is presumed on the basis of calculated GFR or clearance. For drugs with significant clearances on RRT, extra dosing is provided posthemodialysis. However, careful attention is required when we have to administer drugs with predominant renal clearance, nephrotoxicity, and narrow therapeutic index. In this chapter, we will review factors affecting drug dosing, methods of calculating loading and maintenance dose, and few examples of antimicrobial dosing on RRT.

## FACTORS AFFECTING DRUG DOSING (TABLE 1)

### Drug Factors

- *Volume of distribution (VD)*: It is a theoretical volume through which the drug is distributed if the concentration throughout that volume is same as plasma (equilibrium state). Loading dose of antibiotic will depend on VD. Once a drug is administered, the initial fall in drug level is due to this redistribution of the drug and the subsequent fall is due to elimination. The appropriate loading or initial dose of a drug will depend predominantly on VD. Time to equilibration/redistribution across different compartments will depend on drugs physicochemical properties. Maintenance dosages will be determined mainly by time to steady state concentration (4 ½ half-lives) and the rate of elimination of the drug.
- *Solubility*: Hydrophilic antibiotics will have lower VD, low intracellular penetration, and predominantly renal clearance. Lipophilic antibiotic will have larger VD, good intracellular penetration, and predominantly hepatic clearance.

**Table 1:** Factors affecting drug dosing on renal replacement therapy.

| *Factors* | |
|---|---|
| Drug factors | • Volume of distribution (VD)<br>• Hydrophilic or lipophilic<br>• Protein binding<br>• Pharmacokinetic properties<br>• Active metabolites<br>• Clearance |
| Patient factors | • Changes in VD<br>• Changes in protein binding<br>• Residual renal function<br>• Augmented renal clearance |
| Dialysis factors | • Dialysis modality—Timing<br>• Mechanism of solute transfer<br>• Membrane characteristic's<br>• Drug factors (molecular size, protein binding, and drug membrane interactions)<br>• Dialysis prescription factors (blood flow, ultrafiltration, and replacement) |

- *Protein binding*: Higher the protein binding, more is the drug in central compartment and lesser is the VD.
- *Pharmacokinetic properties*: PK of antibiotics such as concentration dependent ($C_{max}$/MIC) or time dependent (T > MIC) or concentration with time-dependent killing (AUC/MIC).
- *Clearance*: Volume of plasma that is completely cleared of drug per unit time. Renal clearance mechanisms include glomerular filtration, tubular reabsorption, and secretion. Nonrenal clearance mechanisms will also be affected either due to associated organ dysfunctions or upregulation of nonrenal clearance. Active metabolites may contribute to some therapeutic effect and/or toxicity.

## Patient Factors

The above PK properties of drugs are significantly affected in critically ill patients. We need to consider patient factors.

- *Volume of distribution*: VD is large in critically ill patients due to poor elimination, fluid retention, third spacing, and also therapeutic fluid administration.
- *Protein binding*: Decrease in protein binding is seen in critically ill patients with associated hypoalbuminemia, changes in pH, and uremia. Hypoalbuminemia > 2.5 mg/DL will affect PK of protein bind drugs.
- *Residual renal function estimation*: Residual renal clearance can be estimated from creatinine clearance (CrCL) equations. Equations for estimation of CrCL like Cockcroft and Gault or MDRD (modification of diet in renal disease) are evaluated for chronic kidney disease. In critically ill patients, due to above mentioned factors, these assumptions may not hold true. To assess kidney functions, more accurate tools like estimated CrCL or estimated GFR or (eGFR) measured GFR should be used. CrCL should be measured, rather than estimated from equations.

- *Augmented clearance*: Hyperdynamic state in critically ill patients increases both renal and hepatic blood flow causing augmented clearance. This can be estimated by timed urinary CrCL. Augmented clearance is seen in young age, lower severity of illness, and higher cardiac index (hyperdynamic septic shock, pregnancy, and anemia). Plasma creatinine-based equations like MDRD, cockcroft gault (CG) does not take in to account augmented clearance.

## Dialysis Factors

### Dialysis Modality

*Timing*: Intermittent vs. Continuous.

Drugs are distributed in central/plasma compartment and tissue compartment. Extracorporeal removal depends on central compartment clearance and rate of transfer (equilibration) between central and tissue compartments. In intermittent hemodialysis (IHD), rate of removal exceeds intercompartmental transfer. In continuous HD, VD will have less impact on drug removal as there is continuous re-equilibration between different compartments. Drug clearance on sustained low-efficiency daily dialysis (SLEDD) is not investigated. As dialysate flows are typically lower in SLEDD (100 mL/min), equilibration of solute levels across blood and dialysate is near complete and clearance will approximate as that of continuous renal replacement.

*Mechanism of solute transfer*: Diffusion or Convection.

On HD, solute clearance is through diffusion of solutes and drugs from high to low concentration across a semipermeable membrane. Molecular weight (MW) of solute, composition of dialysate, and the duration of dialysis treatment affect solute/drug clearance. Only small molecules (<500 Da) are cleared by diffusion. Dialysate flow rates will affect drug clearance. Increasing blood and dialysate flows will initially increase solute clearance but with a ceiling effect. At high blood and dialysate (500–800 mL/min) flow rates used for intermittent dialysis the saturation coefficient ($S_d$) may be lower than for continuous HD due to inadequate time for complete equilibration

In hemofiltration, movement of solutes across membrane is by convection and is under pressure. It effectively clears solutes up to 50,000 Da. Large volume of ultrafiltration formed in this process necessitates replacement.

In hemodiafiltration simultaneous diffusion with convection and ultrafiltration is done leading to better clearance of small, middle, and large molecules.

### Membrane Characteristics

Drug clearance is directly proportional to surface area of membrane (0.5–2.5 $m^2$). Old cellulose or cellophane membranes had pore size of less than 1,000 Da. Biosynthetic membranes like polysulfone, polyacrylonitrile or polyamide typically have pore size 5,000 to 20,000 Da. Drug removal by hemofiltration (convective process) does not depend on molecular size as most antibiotics have smaller MW.

Sieving coefficient ($S_c$) is the ratio of ultrafiltrate concentration to plasma concentration and is between 0 and 1. $S_c$ mostly depends on drugs MW and protein binding. Most antimicrobials have MW of 1,000 Da or less. Glycopeptides like teicoplanin and vancomycin are relatively large drug molecules approximately 1,400–1,800 Da. $S_c$ also depends on membrane types (pore size, surface area) and drug membrane interactions like adsorption and drug charge effect. Adsorption of drugs like aminoglycoside to polyacrylonitrile membrane increases drug clearance, but this adsorption process saturates as duration of dialysis is extended. Drug charge effect (Gibbs Donnan effect) may be significant in clearance of polycationic drugs. Due to inability in clearing of large anionic molecules like albumin (100,000 Da), blood side of membrane is negatively charged and may affect transmembrane clearance of polycationic drugs. Thus phenomenon is reported with aminoglycosides. Modern biosynthetic membranes have pore size of 5,000-20,000 Da facilitating diffusive clearance of small molecules. Continuous renal replacement therapy (CRRT) filters have high pore size and are effective in removing molecules up to 50,000 Da.

### *Dialysis Prescription Factors*

Typically, dialysis prescriptions include modality, duration, blood flows, dialysate flows [for HD and continuous venovenous hemodiafiltration (CVVHDF)], ultrafiltration rate, replacement fluid, replacement fluid location (per or post filter), and anticoagulation. $S_d$ reflects the ability of drug to diffuse across membrane and is expressed as ratio of drug concentration in dialysate to drug concentration in plasma. With high blood and dialysate flows used for IHD, $S_d$ may be low than continuous HD due to inadequate time for equilibration. In SLEDD, this equilibration is nearly complete and $S_d$ approaches to those for CRRT. In addition to membrane characteristics, dialysate flow rate ($Q_d$) and blood flow rate ($Q_b$) will determine the $S_d$. In CRRT, ultrafiltration rate ($Q_f$) or effluent volume is the most important variable in CRRT affecting drug elimination. Composition of dialysis fluid will determine gradient for diffusion in HD.

In case of hemofiltration, location of replacement fluid either prefilter or postfilter also affects drug clearance. Prefilter replacement also known as predilution, results in decreased concentration of solute/drug presented to hemofilter and reduced clearance. This effect will be significant if replacement volumes are high.

## DOSING ON RENAL REPLACEMENT THERAPY

Appropriately dosing an antibiotic to achieve therapeutic levels is important as subtherapeutic levels will not achieve necessary kill.

Drug dosing predominantly depends on VD, drug properties, and total drug clearance. Total drug clearance is effectively a sum of residual renal clearance, clearance by RRT and nonrenal, non-RRT clearance mechanisms.

Changes in physicochemical properties of drugs as well as the pathophysiological changes due to disease seen in critically ill patients make drug dosing difficult. Most PK/PD evaluations for drugs are done on healthy volunteers and their use for calculating dose in critically ill may not hold true.

Most published data related to drug dosing in RRT is related to CRRT.

### Loading Dose

Main determinant of loading dose is VD. Unless the VD is decreased in conditions like severe dehydration, the initial dose of the drug should not be reduced. In most critically ill patients,

VD is significantly increased (e.g. sepsis), warranting a loading dose (D) to achieve a target concentration (C). Mathematically, it can be derived as:

$$D = C \times VD$$

Volume of distribution is mostly derived in healthy population. Also target concentration at site of action may be different from plasma concentrations.

As clearance of renally excreted drugs is also reduced, half-life increases. Steady state concentration of drug which determines therapeutic effect, will be reached later. This warrants against reducing loading dose.

## Maintenance Doses

Options for estimating appropriate maintenance doses:

- Use product insert or published recommendations
- Use a formula
- Use recommendation from primary research paper, checking the results are valid and applicable to our patient
- Derive a dose from first principles and published PK data.

### *Product Insert or Published Recommendations*

Though commonly used, these recommendations are often based on patients with CKD and do not take into consideration issues of critically ill patient or dialysis.

### *Formulae*

A number of formulae have been published and are listed in Table 2.

**Table 2:** Formula for calculating an appropriate dose depending on mode of renal replacement therapy (RRT).

| *Sr. No.* | *Mode of CRRT* | *Formula* |
|---|---|---|
| 1. | CVVH | $D = C_{ss} \times UBF \times Q_f \times I$ |
| 2. | CVVHDF | $D = \frac{D_N (P_x + (1\text{-}P_x)\, Cl_{CRtot})}{Cl_{CRn}}$ |
| 3. | CVVH | $D = \frac{D_N\, [(Cl_{NR} + (Q_f \times S_c)\,]}{Cl_N}$ |
| 4. | All modes | $D = \frac{D_{anuria}}{1\text{-}\left(\frac{Cl_{EC}}{Cl_{EC} + Cl_{NR} + CL_R}\right)}$ |

($Cl_{CRn}$: normal creatinine clearance; $Cl_{CRtot}$: renal + extracorporeal creatinine clearance; $Cl_{EC}$: extracorporeal clearance; $Cl_N$: normal drug clearance; $Cl_{NR}$: nonrenal drug clearance; $Cl_R$: renal clearance; $D_{anuria}$: recommended dose for anuric patients; $D_N$: normal dose; I: dosing interval; $P_x$: extrarenal clearance fraction (= nonrenal, non-RRT drug clearance/normal clearance); $Q_f$: ultrafiltration rate; $S_c$: sieving coefficient; UBF: unbound fraction; CVVH: continuous venovenous hemofiltration; CVVHDF: continuous venovenous hemodiafiltration)

**Table 3:** Formulae for calculating drug clearance by different modes of continuous renal replacement therapy.

| *Mode of CRRT* | *Formula for calculating drug CRRT drug clearance* |
|---|---|
| CVVH predilution | $Cl_{CVVH(pre)} = \dfrac{Q_f \times S_c \times Q_b}{Q_b + Q_{rep}}$ |
| CVVH postdilution | $Cl_{CVVH(post)} = Q_f \times S_c$ |
| CVVHD | $Cl_{CVVHD} = Q_d \times S_d$ |
| CVVHDF | $Cl_{CVVHD} = (Q_f + Q_d) \times S_d$ |

(CRRT: continuous renal replacement therapy; CVVH: continuous venovenous hemofiltration; CVVHD: continuous venovenous hemodialysis; CVVHDF: continuous venovenous hemodiafiltration).

These formulae make a number of assumptions about proportion of free/bound form of drug, known steady state concentrations, no residual renal clearance, and none have been extensively validated.

### Recommendation from Primary Research Paper

It is important to check that the study included critically ill patients with acute renal failure and the renal replacement specifications, residual renal clearance, and the target drug concentration is similar to our patient.

### First Principle

This process involves calculating maintenance dose.

*Steps:*

1. Obtain published PK data from similar critically ill patients with AKI on RRT.
2. Look at data for VD, $S_c$ or $S_d$, and nonrenal, non-RRT clearance.
3. Calculate RRT clearance using formulae for specific modality used (Table 3).
4. Estimate residual renal clearance.
5. Calculate total drug clearance which is sum of RRT, residual renal, and non-RRT, nonrenal clearance.
6. For continuous IV infusion the maintenance dose is:

   Infusion rate = Target concentration × total clearance

   *For IV bolus:*

   Dose = Target concentration × dosing interval × clearance
7. The calculation can be modified for antibiotic dosing so that specific PK targets can be reached.

## FIRST PRINCIPLE STEPS

First principle steps have been shown in Flowchart 1.

**Flowchart 1:** Antibiotic dose calculation for critically ill patients receiving continuous renal replacement therapy, based on pharmacokinetic target.

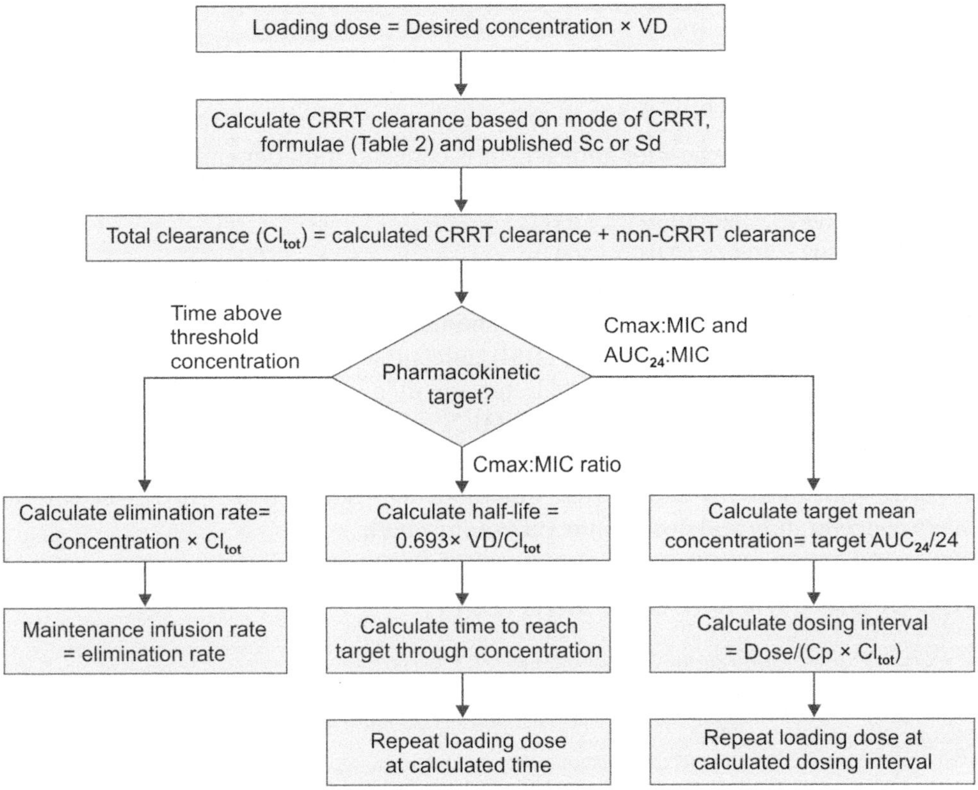


(CRRT: continuous renal replacement therapy; VD: volume of distribution).

## Example of First Principle

A 45-year-old 80 kg patient with end-stage renal failure and septic shock due to hospital-acquired pneumonia is admitted to your intensive care unit (ICU). You decide to give start CVVHDF with total dialysis/effluent of 3 L/hr and to start Amikacin. There is minimal residual renal function.

*Step 1: Loading dose*—depends on VD and desired concentration.

D = VD × Desired concentration

Volume of distribution of amikacin increased in critically ill septic patients. Literature data VD for Amikacin roughly 0.5 L/kg

Desired concentration = 8–10 × MIC (4 μg/mL or 4 mg/L)

Desired concentration = 32 to 40 mg/L

D = VD × Desired concentration

Dose = 0.5 L/kg × 32 mg/L = 16 mg/kg

*Step 2: Maintenance dose*—Calculate clearance using formulas and data for $S_c$ or $S_d$

Clearance = $S_d$ × dialysis flow rate

CRRT clearance = 0.6 × 3,000 mL/hr = 1,800 mL/hr

Plus

Nonrenal clearance 22 mL/min (eGFR) = 1,320 mL/hr

Total clearance = 3,120 mL/hr

*Step 3: Determining PK target*—for amikacin, it is concentration dependant and is expressed as Cmax/MIC.

So, we will have to calculating $t_{1/2} = 0.693 \times V_d/Cl_{total}$

Half-life = 0.693 × 40 L/3.12 L/hr = 8.9 hr

Decreasing the concentration from 32 mg/L to 2 mg/L = 4 half lives

Therefore, dosing interval should be 4 × 8.9 hours = 36 hours

If daily therapeutic drug monitoring (TDM) concentrations are taken, may delay dose by 12 hours or more. If drug is given after 24 hours and then levels checked, may overdose.

For drugs with time-dependent killing (T > MIC), calculate elimination rate = concentration* clearance. Maintenance dose will be equal to elimination rate.

For drugs with both concentration and time-dependent killing (AUC/MIC), calculate target mean concentration and dosing interval to adjust both.

## KDIGO UPDATE ON DRUG DOSING (2011)

| | *Drug dosing considerations* |
|---|---|
| AKI | 1. The KDIGO AKI, AKIN, RIFLE, or pRIFLE criteria should be prospectively utilized to optimize the identification of patients at highest risk of developing AKI<br>2. High-risk medications, those with known nephrotoxicity, or other potential toxicities associated with supratherapeutic serum concentrations should be identified proactively, for example, computerized order entry, so that the prescribing clinician can closely monitor patient response<br>3. The VD of several medications is dramatically increased in the presence of AKI and thus larger loading doses may need to be administered to avoid subtherapeutic responses due to the achievement of lower than desired serum concentrations<br>4. When possible, therapeutic drug monitoring should be utilized for those medications where serum drug concentrations can be obtained in a clinically relevant time frame<br>5. Trends in renal function indices such as serum creatinine and urine output along with volume status should be utilized to guide drug dosing when rapidly measurable indices are unavailable<br>6. For those medications where therapeutic drug monitoring is not possible, close monitoring of drug pharmacodynamic may prove to be a useful surrogate<br>7. Evaluation of risk for drug-drug and drug-nutrient interactions should be facilitated by incorporating validated electronic drug interaction tools into electronic medical records (EMRs)<br>8. A patient-centered team approach that includes an ICU pharmacist is recommended to prevent medication-related problems and enhance safe and effective medication use<br>9. EMRs should maintain records for discontinued medications for up to 7 days to make it possible to assess potential residual effects on the patient's current condition |

| | *Drug dosing considerations* |
|---|---|
| Hemodialysis | 1. The dose should be given after dialysis to ensure active drug levels until next dosing. Consider a supplementary dose in addition to the dose adjusted to kidney failure after dialysis to replace the fraction removed by dialysis<br>2. The supplementary dose derived from studies of low-flux nonsynthetic membranes should empirically be increased by at least 50% when patients are dialyzed with high-flux synthetic dialyzers<br>3. Extended dialysis regimens with high diffusive membranes have been associated with extensive drug clearances and thus the supplementary dose may need to be increased |
| CRRT/EDD (extended daily dialysis) | 1. End-stage renal disease (ESRD) dosing recommendations should be used only as an initial guide for the initiation of therapy in an AKI patient receiving CRRT when no other information is available<br>2. The existing maintenance dosing recommendations for ESRD patients receiving HD often result in the achievement of subtherapeutic concentrations and treatment failures for patients with severe AKI requiring RRT<br>3. The most effective dosing optimization strategy is to use therapeutic drug monitoring for drugs like aminoglycosides and vancomycin to achieve the desired therapeutic goals. However, very few drugs have clinically useful (quick turnaround time, Food and Drug Administration/European Medicines Agency approved) assays available<br>4. When CRRT or EDD clearance data are available, the current literature, recommendations should be the logical starting dose for therapy. Different treatment intensities for CRRT or EDD result in marked variability in drug removal and thus this literature may not be generalizable across the multiple CRRT and EDD prescriptions that are used in practice<br>5. Another alternative is to calculate the "total creatinine clearance" (CLcr) based on the addition of the patient's residual renal clearance and expected extracorporeal clearance. This value can then be used to estimate a maintenance dosing regimen based on medication dosing guidelines specified for that resultant total CLcr range. Using this method, most drugs will fall in the CLcr 25–50 mL/min range<br>6. A fourth method starts with the dose and dosing interval for a patient with a GFR—10 mL/min (anuric dose), and makes dosage adaptations based on the drug fraction expected to be removed by extracorporeal therapy (FrEC)<br>7. A fifth method starts with a normal dose (Dn) and reduces dose based on normal clearance ($Cl_{norm}$), nonrenal clearance ($Cl_{nonrenal}$), effluent rate ($Q_{eff}$), and sieving coefficient (SC)<br>8. CRRT and EDD education should be an integral part of critical care and nephrology fellowship training programs |

(KDIGO: kidney disease improving global outcome; AKIN: acute kidney injury network).

## FUTURE IS THERAPEUTIC DRUG MONITORING

Therapeutic drug monitoring and adjusting the drug dosage accordingly is going to be the future of drug dosings in chronic kidney disease (CKD) patients. Prospective serum drug concentrations measurement and the subsequent use of sound PK/PD therapeutic drug monitoring approaches are required especially for drugs with a narrow therapeutic range. But many a times it is not a possibility due to the unavailability of rapid specific analytical methods for the determination of serum drug concentrations. There are significant gaps in knowledge of the PK and PD of most drugs in AKI and CKD patients.

So the development of excessive pharmacologic effect or toxicity may be the primary indicator of a need for dosage adjustment. There are currently very limited data to guide drug dosing for AKI or multisystem organ failure (MSOF), multiorgan dysfunction syndrome (MODS) patients receiving one of the multiple variants of RRT and need further research and easy availability of drug monitoring tests.

## SUMMARY

- Drugs to be efficacious need to have therapeutic plasma concentration and critical illness mainly renal dysfunction significantly affects the PK and PDs of drugs.
- While considering the drug dosing there are drug factors, patient factors, and dialysis factors all should be taken into consideration.
- There are different considerations in calculating loading dose and maintenance dose as per the first principle.
- Based on understanding of principles of drug removal by CRRT, individual antibiotic dosage and dosing interval may be estimated by mathematical equation.
- Updates for drug dosings in AKI, IHD, and CRRT are available and are getting revised as per ongoing research.
- Therapeutic drug monitoring is going to be the future of clinical practice in this field.

## SUGGESTED READING


1. Brater DC. Drug dosing in patients with impaired renal function. Clin Pharmacol Ther. 2009;86(5):483-9.
2. Clark WR, Hamburger RJ, Lysaght MJ. Effect of membrane composition and structure on solute removal and biocompatibility in hemodialysis. Kidney Int. 1999;56:2005-15.
3. Gabardi S, Abramson S. Drug dosing in chronic kidney disease. Med Clin North Am. 2005;89:649-87.
4. Matzke GR, Comstock T. Influence of renal disease and dialysis on pharmacokinetics. In: Evans W, Schentag J, Burton M (Eds). Applied Pharmacokinetics: Principles of Therapeutic Drug Monitoring, 4th edition. Lippincott, Williams & Wilkins: Baltimore, MD; 2005. pp. 187-212.
5. Matzke GR, George R. Drug dosing consideration in patients with acute and chronic kidney disease, a clinical update from Kidney Disease. Kidney Int. 2011;80(11):1122-37.
6. Munar MY, Singh H. Drug dosing adjustments in patients with chronic kidney disease. Am Fam Physician. 2007;75:1487-96.
7. Murphy JE. Clinical Pharmacokinetics Pocket Reference, 4th edition. American Society of Health-System Pharmacists: Bethesda, MD; 2008.
8. Schetz M. Drug dosing in continuous renal replacement therapy: general rules. Curr Opin Crit Care. 2007;13:645-51.
9. Udy AA, Roberts JA, Boots RJ, et al. Augmented renal clearance: implications for antibacterial dosing in the critically ill. Clin Pharmacokinet. 2010;49:1-16.

CHAPTER 15

# Renal Replacement Therapy in Hepatorenal Syndrome

*Rajasekara Chakravarthi M, Vijay Varma P, Jyothsna G*

## INTRODUCTION

Patients with decompensated cirrhosis of liver are at increased risk of acute kidney injury (AKI) which results in increased morbidity and mortality. It occurs in 25–50% of these patients admitted to the hospital. Hepatorenal syndrome (HRS) accounts for 15–20% of AKI in cirrhotics. The understanding of HRS has changed in the recent years and the concept that HRS is not purely functional in nature is emerging. In addition to renal hypoperfusion due to macrocirculatory dysfunction (i.e. splanchnic arterial vasodilation and reduction of cardiac output), the new theory is that the increased circulating levels of proinflammatory cytokines and chemokines may contribute to the pathophysiology of HRS. The kidneys can be subject to many other insults such as hypovolemia, sepsis-related tubular injury, bile cast nephropathy, and drug-induced renal injury, together now referred to as *non-HRS AKI.*[1]

The prognosis of patients with cirrhosis who develop AKI varies based on the etiology of AKI. Data from the liver group from Barcelona has shown that the 3-month probability of survival was 76% for parenchymal renal disease, 46% for hypovolemia-related AKI, 31% for sepsis-related AKI, and only 15% for patients with HRS.[2]

Renal replacement therapy (RRT) in HRS is controversial and it has been observed that critically ill liver cirrhotic patients requiring RRT have very high mortality independent of liver transplantation (LT) options. Wong et al. studied 102 liver transplant candidates receiving RRT for AKI. A total of 32 (31%) survived to transplant, with 1-year postoperative survival of 70% versus 90% for patients not requiring RRT. Mortality in those not receiving a transplant was near universal, 64/69 (94%).[3] Hence, when attempting to decide whether to propose dialysis in a patient with cirrhosis and AKI, clinicians should be able to answer whether it will help as a bridge to LT or is it going to be a futile attempt resulting in further financial burden to the family.

## INDICATIONS FOR RRT IN HRS

Renal replacement therapy can be considered in nonresponders to vasoconstrictors (Terlipressin, noradrenaline, and midodrine in combination with intravenous albumin).

The indications for RRT in HRS are not different from those for other patients with AKI, i.e. volume overload, refractory metabolic acidosis, uremic complications, and electrolyte disorders such as hyperkalemia.

However, given the poor prognosis in these patients, most clinicians reserve RRT for those patients who are considered candidates for liver transplant or who are being evaluated for LT.[4]

## CHOICE OF RRT MODALITY

Basic techniques that can be used in patients with HRS are:

- Intermittent hemodialysis (IHD) lasting 3–4 hours
- Continuous renal replacement therapies (CRRTs) that last 24 hours/day, such as continuous venovenous hemofiltration (CVVHF), hemodiafiltration (CVVHDF), or hemodialysis (CVVHD)
- Sustained low-efficiency dialysis (SLED), which usually takes 8–12 hours.

The choice of RRT modality should be individualized based on patient's clinical condition as dictated by hemodynamic stability and severity of illness.

Continuous renal replacement therapy may be better tolerated than IHD in terms of:

- Better cardiovascular stability
- More gradual correction of hyponatremia (necessary to avoid central pontine myelinolysis)
- Less fluctuation in intracranial pressure (ICP).

Patients undergoing IHD have episodes of severe hypotension in the first phase of the procedure and progressive ICP elevation by as much as 60% at the end (Fig. 1). The reasons for this could be:

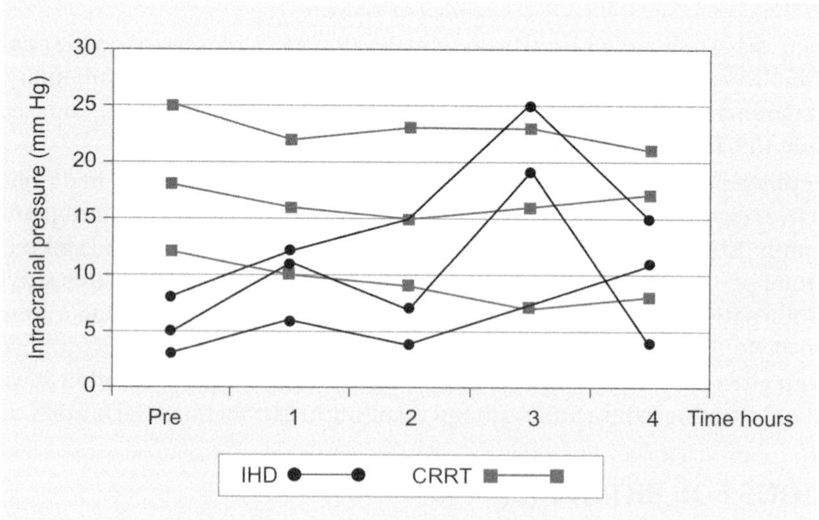


**Fig. 1:** Changes in mean intracranial pressure during intermittent hemodialysis (IHD) and continuous venovenous hemodiafiltration (CVVHDF).
(CRRT: continuous renal replacement therapy)

- Rapid decline in serum osmolality within the first hour of IHD, almost reaching 6 mOsm/kg $H_2O$. In IHD, blood flows at a rate of 250 mL/min and contacts with a large volume of dialysate, which flows at a rate of 500 mL/min, resulting in a high transmembrane gradient with massive diffusion of urea and other osmotically active substances. However, although small molecules quickly pass from extracellular spaces into the dialysate, diffusion from intracellular into extracellular spaces occurs at much slower rates. This results in a transient, relative hyperosmolality of the intracellular compartment and a reversal of water influx into brain cells, leading to a rise in ICP on one hand, and hypovolemia associated with hypotonia on the other.
- Rapid infusion of supraphysiological bicarbonate concentrations during hemodialysis rapidly corrects plasma pH. Bicarbonate is charged and cannot readily cross the blood-brain barrier (BBB). However bicarbonate forms $H_2CO_3$ by reacting with hydrogen ions, which can dissociate into water and carbon dioxide, and carbon dioxide can readily cross the BBB. These fluxes of $HCO_3$, $H_2CO_3$, and carbon dioxide lead to changes in pH according to the Henderson–Hasselbalch equation and result in what is termed a "paradoxical" intracellular acidosis. This then leads to a compensatory production of so called intracellular osmoles and water movement into the brain along a concentration gradient.
- Intradialytic hypotension, which is relatively common during IHD, causes a reduction in cerebral perfusion pressure, with a consequent increase in ICP, due to compensatory cerebral vasodilatation.

In CRRT, the decrease in serum osmolality is gradual and prolonged and greater cardiovascular stability allows for better ICP control.

Hepatorenal syndrome is usually associated with chronic hyponatremia. In these patients, the brain loses not only sodium ions, but also other osmotically active organic molecules, which are supposed to balance the decrease in osmolality of the extracellular fluid. In IHD, rapid correction of hyponatremia takes place and the extracellular environment suddenly becomes hypertonic to the brain, which causes its rapid dehydration and may lead to myelinolysis[5] (Fig. 2).

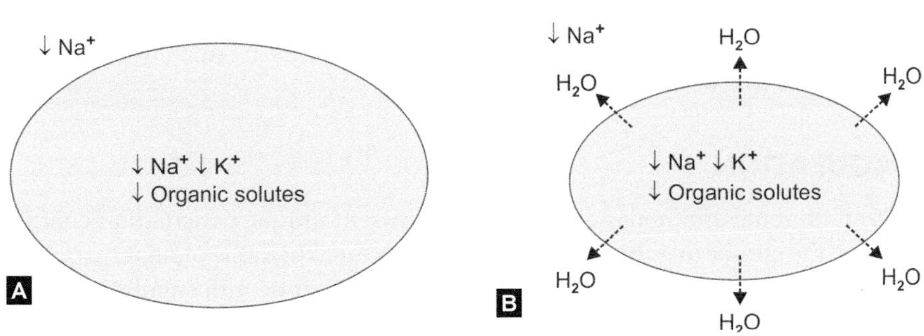


**Figs. 2A and B:** (A) In chronic hyponatremia, the brain loses osmotically active molecules, which is supposed to balance the reduction in osmolality of extracellular fluid and prevent cellular edema; (B) As sodium level is rapidly corrected, increasing hypertonicity of the extracellular fluid leads to sudden dehydration of cells, including brain cells, which may cause myelinolysis.

Continuous renal replacement therapy also has the potential advantage of removing inflammatory cytokines such as TNF-α and IL-6, which have been implicated in the development of AKI and HRS. Despite these presumed advantages, there have been no controlled trials which demonstrate that either modality is superior in HRS.

One clear indication for CRRT is fulminant hepatic failure. Increased intracranial pressure is the most common cause of death in these patients. Therefore, all patients with fulminant hepatic failure should be treated with CRRT.

## ROLE OF INTRAOPERATIVE CRRT DURING LT

Adverse intraoperative hemodynamic events are often seen during the liver transplant surgery. Cross clamping of the inferior vena cava and portal vein during hepatectomy (the an-hepatic phase) reduces the venous return and the cardiac output by 40–50%. Sometimes an extracorporeal circuit (venovenous bypass) can be used to return blood from the infrahepatic inferior vena cava and from the splanchnic circulation to the heart which limits the fall in cardiac output by 20–30%. Following completion of the portal anastomosis, portal unclamping results in large amounts of desaturated blood, potassium, and lactic acid entering the main circulation inducing hypotension, hyperkalemia, and metabolic acidosis, which is described as the "postreperfusion syndrome". Fatal intraoperative ventricular fibrillation from hyperkalemia has been reported during LT. Intraoperative CRRT is feasible and is useful in providing negative or even fluid balance despite a large number of blood transfusions. In addition, it is beneficial in managing hyperkalemia and metabolic acidosis, both of which are common during LT surgery.[4]

## CHOICE OF DIALYSATE

In severe liver dysfunction, metabolism of lactate and acetate to bicarbonate may be impaired, thus a dialysate containing bicarbonate is preferred.

## TIMING OF RRT

The ideal timing for RRT initiation has not been defined in cirrhotic patients with HRS. However, data on AKI in patients with acute liver failure as well as in critically ill patients without liver disease suggest that early RRT improves survival.

## ANTICOAGULATION

Patients with both renal and hepatic impairments present unique coagulation characteristics that complicate the choice of anticoagulation therapies for CRRT. Use of heparin poses a risk of gastrointestinal bleeding, and conducting the procedure without anticoagulation is associated with risk of the filter clotting. The other methods of anticoagulation in this population are:

- *Saline flushes and pre-dilution*: Saline flushes can be infused every 30–60 minutes in the circuit in an attempt to decrease filter clotting. This method is simple and relatively safe but has not been studied extensively. Pre-dilution has been postulated to decrease filter clotting by reducing blood viscosity with the infusion of substitution fluid before the filter.

- *Regional citrate anticoagulation (RCA)*: Another possibility, which has emerged as a promising method in critically ill patients with high risk of bleeding, is regional anticoagulation with citrate, which, leading to depletion of ionized calcium by chelation, interrupts the clotting cascade at several stages. In patients with severe liver failure, citrate metabolism to bicarbonate is significantly impaired, with the risk of citrate accumulation and toxicity, which can result in systemic hypercalcemia, ionized hypocalcemia, and high anion gap metabolic acidosis due to accumulation of citrate and incapacity of the liver to metabolize it into bicarbonate. However, recent data has proven that RCA is a safe and promising alternative even in critically ill liver failure patients suggesting that an extrahepatic metabolism of citrate may exist.[6] The effects of citrate accumulation are not as severe as perceived. The total calcium to ionized calcium ratio ≥2.5 should prompt discontinuation of citrate anticoagulation as it is typically associated with citrate accumulation.

## OTHER EXTRACORPOREAL TECHNIQUES (LIVER DIALYSIS)

In addition to IHD and CRRT, there are several other extracorporeal techniques which have been tried for treatment of both liver and renal failure in cirrhotic patients. These systems consist of membranes and adsorbent-based systems to provide detoxification and dialytic support as well as cell-based systems to provide the excretory, synthetic, and metabolic functions of the liver.

### Molecular Adsorbent Recirculating System

The Molecular Adsorbent Recirculating System (MARS) is designed to remove albumin-bound toxins by albumin dialysis as well as providing standard CRRT. The albumin dialysate is then regenerated utilizing an anion exchange resin and active charcoal adsorption. MARS has been utilized in treatment of HRS and was shown to be superior to CRRT in terms of patient survival and to improve hemodynamics and urine output.

### Prometheus

It employs fractional plasma separation and adsorption with hemodialysis which could be utilized to treat liver failure patients who have a need for RRT.

In two controlled studies, both MARS or Prometheus showed promising, beneficial effects in patients with HRS-AKI, but should be further investigated.[7,8]

## LIVER TRANSPLANTATION AND SIMULTANEOUS LIVER-KIDNEY TRANSPLANTATION

The best therapeutic option in patients with HRS is LT. However, several studies have shown that serum creatinine after LT is higher in patients transplanted with HRS, compared to those without HRS at the time of LT.

Simultaneous liver-kidney transplantation (SLK) can be indicated in patients with *cirrhosis and chronic kidney disease* in the following conditions:

- Estimated GFR (using MDRD6 equation) ≤40 mL/min or measured GFR using iothalamate clearance ≤30 mL/min
- Proteinuria ≥2 g/day
- Kidney biopsy showing >30% global glomerulosclerosis or >30% interstitial fibrosis
- Inherited metabolic disease.

Simultaneous liver–kidney transplantation is also indicated in patients with *cirrhosis and sustained AKI* irrespective of its type, including HRS-AKI when refractory to drug therapy, in the following conditions:

- AKI on RRT for ≥4 weeks
- Estimated GFR ≤35 mL/min or measured GFR ≤25 mL/min ≥4 weeks.[9]

## ROLE OF ASCITIC FLUID ULTRAFILTRATION AND REINFUSION THERAPY

Patients with decompensated cirrhosis have refractory ascites which results in raised intra-abdominal pressure which itself is a risk factor for AKI. Repeated large volume paracentesis (LVP) results in increased risk of peritonitis and also hepatic encephalopathy. Percutaneously placed Tenckhoff peritoneal dialysis (PD) catheter is used to remove the ascitic fluid and then this fluid is passed through the hemodialysis pump and filter for ultrafiltration (Fig. 3). In ascitic fluid ultrafiltration and reinfusion therapy (AURT), albumin which is returned after ultrafiltration is conserved in the body unlike in LVP where it is lost after each session and requires albumin infusion during each session. Piyush et al. have proved that albumin concentrated in the fluid which returns to peritoneal cavity after ultrafiltration moves to portosystemic circulation after few hours, adding to the circulating pool of albumin.[10]

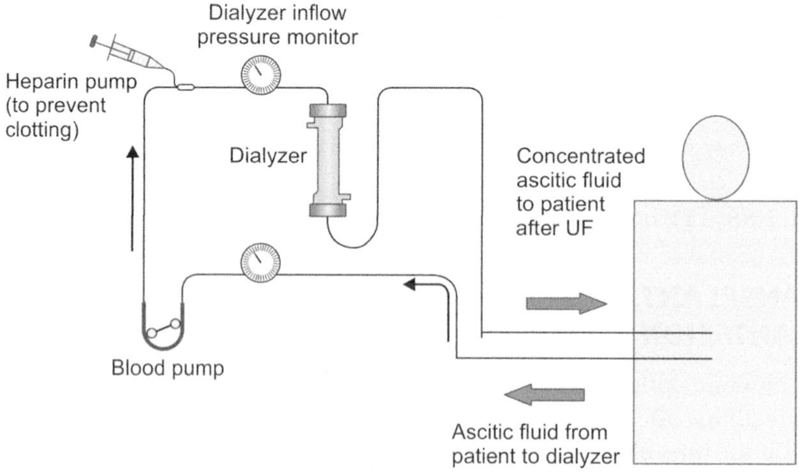


**Fig. 3:** Technique of ascitic fluid ultrafiltration (UF) and reinfusion therapy via percutaneous peritoneal dialysis catheter wherein ascitic fluid is ultrafiltered using hemodialysis filter and then concentrated albumin is reinfused into the peritoneal cavity.

## REFERENCES

1. Davenport A, Sheikh MF, Lamb E, et al. Acute kidney injury in acute-on-chronic liver failure: where does hepatorenal syndrome fit? Kidney Int. 2017;92(5):1058-70.
2. Martin-Llahi M, Guevara M, Torre A, et al. Prognostic importance of the cause of renal failure in patients with cirrhosis. Gastroenterology. 2011;140:488-96.
3. Wong LP, Blackley MP, Andreoni KA, et al. Survival of liver transplant candidates with acute renal failure receiving renal replacement therapy. Kidney Int. 2005;68:362-70.
4. Gonwa TA, Wadei HM. The challenges of providing renal replacement therapy in decompensated liver cirrhosis. Blood Purif. 2012;33(1-3):144-8.
5. Matuszkiewicz-Rowińska J, Wieliczko M, Małyszko J. Renal replacement therapy before, during, and after orthotopic liver transplantation. Ann Transplant. 2013;18:248-55.
6. Zhang W, Bai M, Yu Y, et al. Safety and efficacy of regional citrate anticoagulation for continuous renal replacement therapy in liver failure patients: a systematic review and meta-analysis. Crit Care. 2019;23(1):22.
7. Banares R, Nevens F, Larsen FS, et al. Extracorporeal albumin dialysis with the molecular adsorbent recirculating system in acute-on-chronic liver failure: the RELIEF trial. Hepatology. 2013;57:1153-62.
8. Kribben A, Gerken G, Haag S, et al. Effects of fractionated plasma separation and adsorption on survival in patients with acute-on-chronic liver failure. Gastroenterology. 2012;142:782-9.
9. Angeli P, Bernardi M, Villanueva C, et al. EASL Clinical Practice Guidelines for the management of patients with decompensated cirrhosis. J Hepatol. 2018;69(2):406-60.
10. Mathur P, Chakravarthi R, Babu S, et al. Ascitic Fluid Ultrafiltration and Reinfusion Therapy (AURT). 2014;4(2):45-6.

CHAPTER 16

# Extracorporeal Therapies in Sepsis: An Update

*Ranajit Chatterjee, Ashutosh Garg*

## INTRODUCTION

Sepsis is one of the leading causes of morbidity and mortality worldwide. The definition of sepsis has evolved over the years. An older definition was based on systemic inflammatory response syndrome (SIRS) criteria. In newer definition of sepsis 3.0 (2016), SIRS was replaced with the quick Sequential Organ Failure Assessment score (qSOFA). Now sepsis is a dysregulated immune response to infections that results in life-threatening organ dysfunction.

Richard Pfeiffer discovered that a toxic substance associated with bacterial membrane and called it "endotoxin".[1] Endotoxin infusion mimics inflammatory, metabolic, and cardiovascular changes observed in sepsis patients and represents one of the main inducers of shock in sepsis. The discoverer of its receptor (the Toll-like receptor 4),[2] Nüsslein Volhard, was awarded the Nobel prize for this discovery in 1995. Clinical research has shown that endotoxin is indeed circulating in the blood of up to 50% of septic shock patients[3] and associated with poor clinical outcome.[4] In view of the important role of endotoxin in sepsis patients, the idea of "blood purification" emerged.

Bacterial cell wall components (endotoxin or lipopolysaccharide), known as pathogen-associated molecular patterns (PAMPs), as well as damage-associated molecular patterns (DAMPs) released by host injured cells, are well-recognized triggers resulting in the elevation of both pro-inflammatory and anti-inflammatory cytokines. Understanding this complex pathophysiology has led to the development of therapeutic strategies aimed at restoring a balanced immune response by eliminating/deactivating these inflammatory mediators. An unregulated and overwhelming response in the presence of severe sepsis is associated with negative outcomes.

Ronco et al.[5] conceived the *peak concentration hypothesis* in which clinicians effort to remove mediators and cytokines from the blood compartment at the pro-inflammatory phase of sepsis. By reducing the amount of free cytokines, it is hoped that the level of remote organ (associated) damages can be dramatically decreased and, as a consequence, the overall death rate. In this regard, it is still not known what will happen at the interstitial and tissue level with regard to mediators and cytokines which are obviously the most important part in terms of consequences at the tissue level. In this setting, techniques that can more rapidly and substantially remove great amounts of cytokines or mediators are privileged. Among these, there is high-volume and very high-volume hemofiltration and a number of hybrid therapies encompassing high-permeability hemofiltration, super high-flux hemofiltration, hemoadsorption or coupled filtration, and adsorption are used normally in hemofiltration-derived techniques.

The second concept is called the *threshold immunomodulation hypothesis*, also called the *Honoré concept*. In this concept, the view of the system is much more dynamic. In experiments when removal is occurring on the blood compartment side, the level on the interstitial side and the tissue side is also changing and, because not only mediators but also pro-mediators are being removed, some pathways have really stopped when enough pro-mediators have been removed by this technique. At this point, the cascade is blocked and this point is called the *threshold point*. At this level, the cascade is lost and no further harm can be done to the tissue of the organism. Obviously, it is difficult to know when this point has been reached once HVHF is applied. But what is known is that hemodynamics and survival can be improved in some patients as shown by various studies using HVHF without any significant drop in mediators inside the blood compartment itself. This effect is obtained without a dramatic fall in the plasma cytokine level because the cytokine or mediator levels should fall at the tissue level and not specifically at the blood compartment level. Nevertheless, the exact mechanism by which HVHF increases the flow of mediators and cytokines between the interstitial compartment and the blood compartment (and back to the blood side) is not known. Before the end of 2005, it was found that this missing step is perhaps well explained by the last theory.

The third theory is called the *mediator delivery hypothesis* and has also been called the *Alexander concept*. In this theory, the use of HVHF and especially high intakes of incoming fluids (3–5 L/hr) is able to increase the lymphatic flow 20- to 40-fold, even more so for mediators and cytokine lymphatic flow (drag). This has been demonstrated by several reports and is obviously extremely important.

Continuous renal replacement therapy (CRRT) is generally reserved for hemodynamically unstable patients in acute kidney injury (AKI) induced by sepsis. Another application for RRT (sp. hemofiltration) is the extracorporeal removal of inflammatory mediators.

## ROLE OF EXTRACORPOREAL THERAPIES IN THE MANAGEMENT OF SEPSIS

Sepsis needs both a strong inflammatory phase for the physiological clearance of infective insults (Fig. 1, Area A) and presumably a counteractive/protective anti-inflammatory phase for immune reconstitution and recovery (Fig. 1, Area C). The goal is to counter the systemic adverse influence of the cytokine storm, which is disproportionate and counterproductive (Fig. 1, Area B). Apart from the lack of a clear target or targets for removal, we have a limited understanding for determining the severity and immune stage of sepsis. An intervention in either the adaptive inflammatory (Phase A) or the immune-recovering anti-inflammatory phase (Phase C) might do more harm than good in these instances. Maximum benefit of ECT is in cytokine storm phase (phase B).

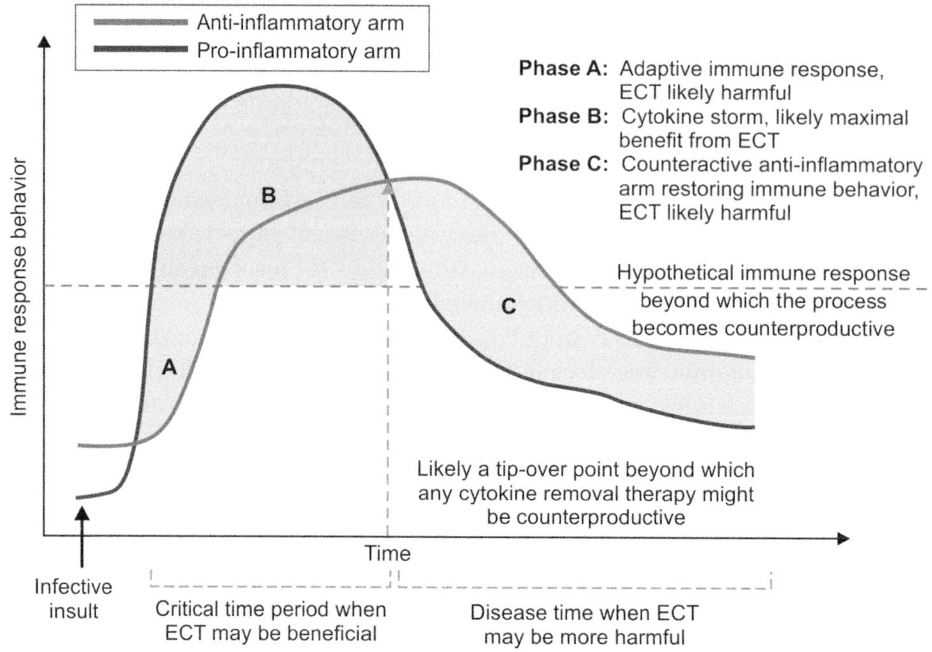


**Fig. 1:** Theoretical considerations of the likely impact of ECT in a single-hit model of sepsis, and its correlation to the stage and severity of disease.
(ECT: extracorporeal therapy) *(For color version, see Plate 6)*

## Major Evolving Therapies

- High-volume hemofiltration and very high-volume hemofiltration
- High cut-off (HCO) membranes
- Adsorption alone
- Coupled plasma filtration adsorption (CPFA).

### *High-volume Hemofiltration and Very High-volume Hemofiltration*

High-volume hemofiltration was defined as continuous treatment with a convective target dose greater than 35 mL/kg/hr. Doses greater than 45 mL/kg/hr were defined as VHVHF. As a technique, it has been utilized for immunomodulation in the context of both AKI[6,7] and sepsis. The largest and only multi-center RCT to date is the IVOIRE trial[8]. It should be noted that different protocols were used with doses ranging from 40 mL/kg/hr to 70 mL/kg/hr. The results overall were inconsistent. Earlier observational studies have suggested a mortality benefit and improvement of hemodynamics, while later studies (IVOIRE trial in particular) did not confirm these findings. In a recent RCT involving a subpopulation of patients with septic shock secondary to burns, HVHF (versus standard therapy) was found to be effective in improving organ function but not survival.[9] To conclude, despite the promising results of earlier studies, HVHF seems to have no significant impact on short-term mortality, improvement in hemodynamics, or reduction in intensive care unit (ICU) or hospital length-of-stay (LOS).

## *High Cut-off Membranes*

High cut-off membranes are characterized by a large pore size [average pore diameter (20 nm) compared with the standard high-flux membrane (10 nm)]. HCO membrane use is similar to the standard RRT prescription, including the choice of anticoagulation. The prescribed dose is typically in the range from 25 mL/kg/hr to 40 mL/kg/hr, as recommended by Kidney Disease Improving Global Outcomes (KDIGO) guidelines. Convective modalities would maximize the HCO membrane ability to remove pro/anti-inflammatory mediators,[10] but the excessive albumin loss commonly observed with the use of such membranes dictates the utilization of only diffusive modalities.

One study comparing continuous venovenous hemodialysis with HCO membranes (HCO-CVVHD; at a dose of 35 mL/kg/hr) vs CVVHDF (at a dose of 45 mL/kg/hr) showed an ICU mortality benefit [37.5% and 87.5% for HCO-CVVHD and CVVHDF groups, respectively ($p = 0.03$)], but no significant difference was found in ICU-LOS and in-hospital mortality.[11] Furthermore, the High Cut-Off Sepsis study (HICOSS) comparing conventional and HCO membranes was stopped prematurely after enrolment of 81 patients due to a lack of 28-day mortality benefit [HCO (31%) vs conventional (33%)] and lack of a difference in vasopressor requirement or ICU-LOS.[12]

## *Adsorption*

Adsorption is performed in the form of hemoperfusion (HP), plasma perfusion, or CPFA. HP involves passage of blood through a hemofilter where mediators are adsorbed to the membrane surface or through a sorbent-containing cartridge. In sepsis, it is generally advocated for treating patients with suspected Gram-negative sepsis or septic shock. Adsorption can be used in isolation or in combination with HD or continuous venovenous hemofiltration (CVVH). More than one session is often required to overcome the possible rebound.

### *Polymyxin B-immobilized Fiber Column (PMX; Toraymyxin)*

*EUPHAS trial*[13] suggested a mortality benefit (28-day mortality, 32% in the treatment group vs 53% in the control group adjusted HR 0.36, 95% CI 0.16–0.80) and a hemodynamic benefit, but no effect on ICU-LOS [20.3 days in PMX group (95% CI 15.0–25.5 days) vs. 18.3 days (95% CI 8.8–27.8 days) in the control group; $p = 0.72$].

*ABDO-MIX trial*[14] suggested no mortality benefit (28-day mortality 27.7% in the treatment group vs. 19.5% in the control group; $p = 0.14$; OR 1.5872; 95% CI 0.8583–2.935) and no impact on hemodynamics or ICU-LOS (11 days in the PMX-HP vs 10 days in the control group; $p = 0.49$). However, cartridge clotting and treatment failure rates were high in this trial (two PMX sessions were completed in only 69.8% of patients), which may partially explain the findings. A recent meta-analysis[15] (seven RCTs, 841 patients) suggested a reduction of mortality (RR 0.65; 95% CI 0.47–0.89; p = 0.007), which was similar to the results of the previous meta-analyses conducted by Cruz et al[16] (RR 0.50; 95% CI 0.37–0.68), Qiu et al.[17] (RR 0.24; 95% CI 0.16–0.38), and Zhou et al.[18] (RR 0.57; 95% CI 0.45- 0.72). However, it was considered to be low-quality evidence due to the serious risk of bias. All the trials were small, open-label, and conducted in single centers in Japan. Additionally, most of the trials involved a surgical population, and thus the results may need to be interpreted with caution when applying the results to medical ICU patients.

*EUPHRATES trial*[19] conducted in North America has recently published results. For blinding purpose patients allocated to polymyxin B hemoperfusion group and control group which received sham hemoperfusion. For sham treatments, a hemodialysis machine was primed at the bedside with a standard bloodline and dialyzer, a dialysis catheter was cut to simulate insertion and taped to the skin beneath an opaque dressing, and 0.9% saline was recirculated in the circuit for 2 hours to simulate a hemoperfusion treatment.

Polymyxin B hemoperfusion was not associated with a significant difference in mortality at 28 days among all participants [treatment group, 84 of 223 (37.7%) vs sham group 78 of 226 (34.5%); risk difference (RD), 3.2%; 95% CI, –5.7% to 12.0%; relative risk (RR), 1.09; 95% CI, 0.85–1.39; $p = 0.49$] or in the population with a Multiple Organ Dysfunction Score (MODS) of more than 9 [treatment group, 65 of 146 (44.5%) vs. sham, 65 of 148 (43.9%); RD, 0.6%; 95% CI, –10.8% to 11.9%; RR, 1.01; 95% CI, 0.78–1.31; $p = 0.92$]. Among patients with septic shock and high endotoxin activity, polymyxin B hemoperfusion treatment plus conventional medical therapy compared with sham treatment plus conventional medical therapy did not reduce mortality at 28 days.

### CytoSorb

The evidence for CytoSorb is limited to case reports/series and a few RCTs, but it is growing. Observational data suggest improvement in hemodynamics and a trend toward decreased mortality. A clinical registry on the use of CytoSorb involving 22 countries has been developed, and according to its most recent report, the use of CytoSorb in 135 septic patients was not associated with side effects. The observed mortality was 65% compared with a predicted risk of death of 78% based on the Acute Physiology and Chronic Health Evaluation II (APACHE II) score. A marked reduction of IL-6 levels was also observed.[20] One drawback is that CytoSorb does not capture endotoxins and IL-10. Another caveat is the treatment duration (average 191 ± 56 minutes compared with treatment lasting for up to 7 days in other studies). This emphasizes the effect of both the initial level of cytokines and the treatment frequency/duration on the extent of cytokine reduction.

### HA-330

Two small RCTs described effectiveness of HA-330 in decreasing inflammatory mediators, along with an improvement in hemodynamics, mortality, and ICU-LOS. One of the trials was conducted in septic patients with acute lung injury, in which there was marked improvement in respiratory parameters in the HP group.[21]

### Modified AN69 (Oxiris)

The evidence supporting the use of modified AN69 is limited to case series. In the study reported by Shum et al.[22] oXiris®-CVVH was delivered to six patients with septic AKI, and the results were compared to 24 severity-matched controls undergoing standard therapy. The results demonstrated that the SOFA score was reduced after 48-h CVVH from the value at

ICU admission by 38% in the oXiris® group, while it was increased by 3% in the control group. No significant difference was observed in ICU and in-hospital mortality between the two groups. More studies investigating its effectiveness are ongoing.

### *LPS Adsorbers (Alteco)*

Evidence for lipopolysaccharide (LPS) adsorbers was obtained from case reports/series that showed a decrease in endotoxin level as well as improvement in patient hemodynamics with no significant side effects. A feasibility study *(ASSET trial)* was unfortunately terminated early due to difficulty recruiting patients.

### *Coupled Plasma Filtration Adsorption*

Coupled plasma filtration adsorption (CPFA™) is a combination of separation of plasma from the cellular components of blood with a highly permeable filter, followed by sorbent adsorption of the plasma component with a styrene resin to remove a number of different cytokines and then reinfusion of the purified plasma before the hemofilter to finally simultaneously provide CRRT for renal/fluid support. The advantage of CPFA is the lack of direct contact between blood cells with the sorbent material, which leads to improved biocompatibility.

A recent meta-analysis that involved 14 studies suggested a potential improvement in survival, but the studies were not high quality and had a small size. The largest RCT to date is the *COMPACT trial*[23] involving 192 patients randomized to either standard of care vs. CPFA plus standard of care. There was no difference in hospital mortality [controls (47.3%) vs CPFA (45.1%); $p = 0.76$] or ICU-free days during the first 30 days (6.8 vs 7.5; $p = 0.35$). The trial was stopped prematurely due to futility. COMPACT I highlighted a few technical issues related to CPFA. First, nearly half of the patients in the CPFA arm did not reach the planned dose. Clotting of the circuit was the cause in 48% of cases despite the use of heparin. Second, cost was a major concern. The high cost contributed to under-treatment, as replacing the circuit when the treatment was interrupted due to clotting was not possible. Finally, CPFA requires adequate staff training because it is somewhat complex. Two other large RCTs are ongoing COMPACT II and ROMPA, which should help expand the body of evidence concerning the feasibility and effectiveness of CPFA.

## ADVERSE EVENTS

Common to all the techniques are extracorporeal circuit-related adverse events. The risks of bleeding, clotting/changes in anticoagulation requirements, drops in platelet counts, and catheter complications are all well-known. Also common to all techniques is the important issue of drug removal. Antimicrobials, in particular, are of utmost importance. In septic patients, antibiotics are the only proven therapy. The risk of antibiotic removal, or under-dosing of patients, should be carefully accounted for by accurate drug level monitoring. In an *in vitro* study examining the effect of adsorption on drug removal,[24] vancomycin, for instance, showed a significant reduction in levels at different time points following adsorption therapy. Additional antibiotics doses may often be required.

An unpredictable loss of beneficial molecules such as albumin (particularly in the case of HCO membrane use), other nutrients, and amino acids is another important consideration. Electrolyte imbalances (hypophosphatemia and hypokalemia in particular) are other important issues that could be harmful, particularly in critically ill patients, and should be carefully monitored. The risk is more pronounced in HVHF use, as emphasized by Clark et al. Frequent monitoring and pre-prepared protocols for electrolyte replacement are important. Finally, all these techniques share the disadvantage of high cost. The current level of evidence is not in favor of utilizing these techniques given the high cost.

As far as technique-specific adverse events, adsorption is associated with thrombocytopenia and leukopenia. HVHF places patients at risk of hemodynamic instability and hypothermia with high convection.[25]

## FUTURE DIRECTIONS

Therapeutic strategies aiming at elimination of the inflammatory mediators involved in the pathogenesis of sepsis represent an attractive and evolving area. Evidence to support ECT use is growing but remains controversial at this stage. There is hemodynamic improvement with different technique of ECT but in terms of decreasing mortality and length of ICU/hospital stay evidences are limited and somewhat conflicting. These techniques may potentially serve as a bridge to stabilize critically ill patients until more definitive therapies take place. Therapy should be tailored to the individual patient condition. The stage at which the patient is captured may influence the choice of modality.

Earlier in the course, when levels of endotoxins and cytokines are extremely high, the application of adsorption/CPFA may help deactivate and decrease the peak elevation of these mediators, resulting in clinical outcomes. Later in the course, adsorption techniques may not be as effective, as the damage caused by the elevated mediators has already taken place, and utilization of the potential benefits of HCO membranes or HVHF for organ support may be more appropriate. Further studies are needed to confirm the theoretical effect of timing of the start of therapy on the utilized modality.

Adsorption, if applied early in the course during which the inflammatory mediator level is at its peak and continued sufficiently long, may represent a more promising tool in comparison to the other techniques. However, this hypothesis remains to be confirmed.

## CONCLUSION

In spite of efforts made to utilize ECT as an effective tool to treat patients of sepsis, evidence is not sufficient enough to support the use of these techniques in sepsis. However, further efforts to try to identify research gaps in an attempt to optimize their use in septic patients are warranted. Our review aims to provide a comprehensive overview concerning both the benefits and risks of these techniques. Further studies to guide clinicians in the application of these techniques in the proper clinical setting are still needed.

## REFERENCES


1. Pfeiffer R. Untersuchungen über das Choleragift. Z Hyg Infektionskr. 1892;11:393-412.
2. Anderson KV, Bokla L, Nusslein-Volhard C. Establishment of dorsal-ventral polarity in the Drosophila embryo: the induction of polarity by the Toll gene product. Cell. 1985;42:791-8.
3. Marshall JC, Walker PM, Foster DM, et al. Measurement of endotoxin activity in critically ill patients using whole blood neutrophil dependent chemiluminescence. Crit Care (Lond). 2002;6:342-8.
4. Opal SM, Scannon PJ, Vincent JL, et al. Relationship between plasma levels of lipopolysaccharide (LPS) and LPS-binding protein in patients with severe sepsis and septic shock. J Infect Dis. 1999;180:1584-9.
5. Ronco C, Bonello M, Bordoni V, et al. Extracorporeal therapies in non-renal disease: treatment of sepsis and the peak concentration hypothesis. Blood Purif. 2004;22:164-74.
6. VA/NIH Acute Renal Failure Trial Network; Palevsky PM, Zhang JH, O'Connor TZ, et al. Intensity of renal support in critically ill patients with acute kidney injury. N Engl J Med. 2008;359(1):7-20.
7. Intensity of continuous renal-replacement therapy in critically ill patients. N Engl J Med. 2009;361(17):1627–38.
8. Joannes-Boyau O, Honoré PM, Perez P, et al. High-volume versus standard-volume haemofiltration for septic shock patients with acute kidney injury (IVOIRE study): a multicentre randomized controlled trial. Intensive Care Med. 2013;39(9):1535-46.
9. Chung KK, Coates EC, Smith DJ, et al. High-volume hemofiltration in adult burn patients with septic shock and acute kidney injury: a multicenter randomized controlled trial. Crit Care. 2017;21(1):4-11.
10. Morgera S, Slowinski T, Melzer C, et al. Renal replacement therapy with high-cutoff hemofilters: impact of convection and diffusion on cytokine clearances and protein status. Am J Kidney Dis. 2004;43(3):444-53.
11. Chelazzi C, Villa G, D'Alfonso MG, et al. Hemodialysis with high cut-off hemodialyzers in patients with multi-drug resistant Gram-negative sepsis and acute kidney injury: a retrospective, case control study. Blood Purif. 2016;42(3):186-93.
12. Honore PM, Clark W. Novel therapeutical concepts for extracorporeal treatment of hyperinflammation and sepsis: immunomodulation. approach with a novel high cut-off membrane: the SepteX membrane. In Proceedings of 10th Congress of World Federation of CCU (WFSICCM) 2009. Florence.
13. Cruz DN, Antonelli M, Fumagalli R, et al. Early use of polymyxin B hemoperfusion in abdominal septic shock: the EUPHAS randomized controlled trial. JAMA. 2009;301(23):2445.
14. Payen DM, Guilhot J, Launey Y, et al. Early use of polymyxin B hemoperfusion in patients with septic shock due to peritonitis: a multicenter randomized control trial. Intensive Care Med. 2015;41:975-84.
15. Kellum JA, Venkataraman R, Powner D, et al. Feasibility study of cytokine removal by hemoadsorption in brain-dead humans. Crit Care Med. 2008;36(1):268-72.
16. Cruz DN, Perazella MA, Bellomo R, et al. Effectiveness of polymyxin B immobilized fiber column in sepsis: a systematic review. Crit Care. 2007;11(2):R47.
17. Qiu XH, Liu SQ, Guo FM, et al. A meta-analysis of the effects of direct hemoperfusion with polymyxin B-immobilized fiber on prognosis in severe sepsis. Zhonghua Nei Ke Za Zhi. 2011;50(4):316-21.
18. Zhou F, Peng Z, Murugan R, et al. Blood purification and mortality in sepsis: a meta-analysis of randomized trials. Crit Care Med. 2013;41(9):2209-20.
19. Iba T, Fowler L. Is polymyxin B-immobilized fiber column ineffective for septic shock? A discussion on the press release for EUPHRATES trial. J Intensive Care. 2017;5:40.
20. Friesecke S, Träger K, Schittek GA, et al. International registry on the use of the CytoSorb® adsorber in ICU patients. Medizinische Klinik-Intensivmedizin und Notfallmedizin; 2017. pp.1-9.

21. Huang Z, Wang SR, Yang ZL, et al. Effect on extrapulmonary sepsis induced acute lung injury by hemoperfusion with neutral microporous resin column. Ther Apher Dial. 2013;17(4):454-61.
22. Shum HP, Chan KC, Kwan MC, et al. Application of endotoxin and cytokine adsorption haemofilter in septic acute kidney injury due to Gram negative bacterial infection. Hong Kong Med J. 2013;19(6):491-7.
23. Livigni S, Bertolini G, Rossi C, et al. Efficacy of coupled plasma filtration adsorption (CPFA) in patients with septic shock: a multicenter randomised controlled clinical trial. BMJ Open. 2014;4(1):e003536.
24. Reiter K, Bordoni V, Dall'Olio G, et al. In vitro removal of therapeutic drugs with a novel adsorbent system. Blood Purif. 2002;20(4):380-8.
25. Rokyta R, Matejovic M, Krouzecky A, et al. Effects of continuous venovenous haemofiltration- induced cooling on global haemodynamics, splanchnic oxygen and energy balance in critically ill patients. Nephrol Dial Transplant. 2004;19(3):623-30.

CHAPTER 17

# Extracorporeal Therapies in Poisoning

*Valentine Lobo*

## INTRODUCTION

The application of extracorporeal therapy is carried out every day to millions of patients with organ failure to remove endogenous toxins not being cleared by the diseased organ. Similarly the application of extracorporeal therapy may be applied to removal of exogenous toxins either accidentally ingested or to which patients may have been exposed. Such application of dialysis to poisoning was in fact done prior to the use of dialysis as renal replacement therapy and is still used in ICUs. However exogenous toxins behave differently from endogenous and their removal by extracorporeal therapies is the focus of this chapter (Box 1).

It must be emphasized that extracorporeal therapy is most often an adjunct and not the primary treatment of poisoning and that all other measures must be simultaneously undertaken.

Several properties determine the extent to which a drug may be removed by an extracorporeal therapy and also the optimal therapy that must be used and these are summarized in Table 1.

## MOLECULAR WEIGHT

Conventional dialysis membranes are high efficiency dialyzers and have a limited pore size. The sieving coefficient drops to 0 at a molecular weight around 10,000 daltons and thus smaller

**Box 1:** Indications for extracorporeal treatment in poisoning.

- Life-threatening toxicity
- Prolonged ICU care and mechanical ventilation
- High likelihood of permanent disability (e.g. blindness following methanol overdose)
- Unavailability of antidote or supportive measures to limit toxicity
- Complications—coma, pneumonia or septicemia or predisposing conditions like chronic obstructive pulmonary disease
- Impaired normal drug excretion—renal, hepatic or cardiac insufficiency
- Metabolic and/or delayed effects (methanol, ethylene glycol, and paraquat)
- All endogenous clearance <4 mL/kg/min
- Volume of distribution <1–2 L/kg
- Narrow therapeutic to toxic index (lithium and digoxin)

**Table 1:** Properties determining toxin removal by extracorporeal therapy.

| *Property of toxin* | *Hemodialysis* | *Hemodiafiltration* | *Hemoperfusion* |
|---|---|---|---|
| Molecular weight (Daltons) | <500 | 500–40,000 | >40,000 |
| Protein binding* | Low | Low | Either |
| Volume of distribution | <1 L/kg | <1 L/kg | <1 L/kg |
| Solubility | Water | Water | Water/Lipid |
| Endogenous clearance | <4 mL/kg/min | <4 mL/kg/min | <4 mL/kg/min |
| Distribution time | Short | Long | Short |

*The product information leaflet will usually provide this information otherwise it may be available from standard pharmacology or toxicology texts.

molecules are removed more efficiently than larger ones. High flux dialyzers offer the possibility of removing larger molecules while recent high cutoff membranes may even remove larger and protein bound toxins. The experience with such dialyzers is limited and the cost generally limits their use.

## PROTEIN BINDING

Toxins in plasma exist in two forms, free and protein bound. Drug removal during dialysis is dependent upon the concentration gradient of unbound (free) drug across the dialysis membrane. Drug albumin complex is often unable to cross the dialysis membrane; hence the ratio of free to albumin bound toxin determines dialytic removal.

## VOLUME OF DISTRIBUTION

A drug with a large volume of distribution (VD) is distributed widely throughout tissues and is present in relatively small amounts in the blood, which is the only part of the total body water accessed by the dialyzer and is likely to be removed. Factors that contribute to a large VD include a high degree of lipid solubility and low plasma protein binding.

## WATER SOLUBILITY

The dialysate used for hemodialysis is aqueous and thus, drugs with high water solubility will be dialyzed more than those with high lipid solubility. Highly lipid-soluble drugs tend to be distributed throughout tissues including those rich in fat, and therefore only a small fraction of the free drug is present in plasma and is accessible for dialysis.

## ENDOGENOUS CLEARANCE

This includes renal, hepatic, and gastrointestinal clearance of the drug.

The use of extracorporeal treatment is justified, if it increases total body clearance by at least 30%.

*A "clinical algorithm" to manage cases of poisoning where specific guidelines are not available runs as follows*:

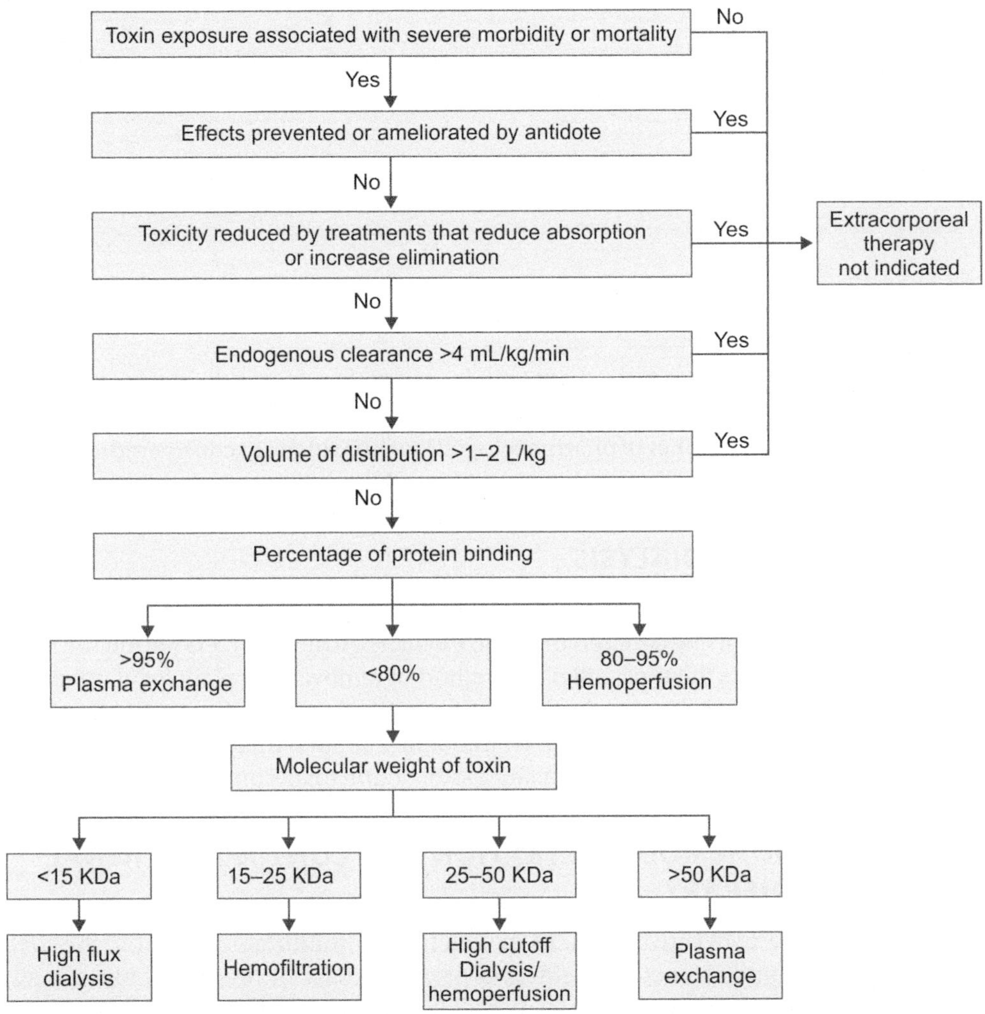


As an example, the use of glucose infusions and continuous or frequent monitoring is easier, less costly, and equally effective in preventing the lethal hypoglycemia with oral antidiabetic drugs than an extracorporeal therapy. In contrast the lactic acidosis that may accompany metformin overdose in a patient with renal impairment or acute kidney injury necessitates hemodialysis slow low-efficiency extended daily dialysis (SLEDD) or even continuous renal replacement therapy (CRRT) early in such cases to avoid fatalities. Similarly activated charcoal to decrease absorption and the use of forced alkaline dieresis in barbiturate overdose may remove the need for extracorporeal therapy.

The use of antidotes like naloxone for opiate overdose and N-acetyl cysteine for paracetamol poisoning are examples of powerful antidotes that render extracorporeal therapy unnecessary.

**Box 2:** List of some poisons lethal to children.

- Calcium antagonists
- Camphor
- Clonidine and other imidazolines
- Lomotil (diphenoxylate/atropine)
- Opiates
- Salicylates
- Sulfonylureas
- Toxic alcohols
- Tricyclic antidepressants

**Box 3:** Pharmacological toxins.

- Ethylene glycol
- Lithium
- Salicylate
- Acetaminophen
- Ethanol
- Methanol
- Metformin
- Benzodiazepines
- Cardiac glycosides
- Calcium channel blockers
- Valproic acid
- Beta adrenergic antagonists
- Atypical antipsychotics
- Methadone
- Oxycodone
- Nonsteroidal anti-inflammatory drugs
- Tricyclic antidepressants
- Cocaine
- Heroin
- Isopropanol

Mention must be made that certain poisons maybe lethal to children even at low doses not otherwise considered toxic (Box 2).

Knowledge of the properties of the toxin and the principles of the individual extracorporeal therapies allows for selection of optimum modalities.

Box 3 shows the small number of pharmacological toxins which are considered amenable to extracorporeal removal in the USA and for which these therapies are most commonly applied.

## INTERMITTENT HEMODIALYSIS

Makes use of diffusion of the toxin across a semipermeable membrane down a concentration gradient into a dialysate flowing countercurrent to blood. High flux dialyzers permit the removal of toxins up to 15 kDa. It is the most efficient method of removal of low molecular toxins and also corrects the acid-base and metabolic derangements that may be associated with poisoning. Being easily available and cheap it is the most frequently applied therapy for poisoning, but a rebound may be seen in the case of protein and tissue bound toxins once the treatment is over.

## HEMOFILTRATION/HEMODIAFILTRATION AND CONTINUOUS RENAL REPLACEMENT THERAPY

These therapies add a convective element in which the ultrafiltrate containing the toxin is replaced by a sterile replacement fluid either in premixed bags or prepared online. It allows removal of larger molecules up to a molecular weight of 25 kDa. A theoretical advantage of CRRT is prevention of a rebound since continuous removal of the toxin although at a very much slower rate compared with intermittent therapies is possible, but the impact of this on clinical outcomes remains unclear.

## HEMOPERFUSION

This requires the passage of blood or separated plasma over a charcoal cartridge which competes with protein for binding high molecular weight toxins. Blood flow requires to be slower and anticoagulation higher than in hemodialysis to increase efficiency. The process is limited by saturation of the cartridge binding sites and the need to replace the cartridge. In addition the cartridge requires frequent replacement and causes loss of leukocytes in 10% and platelets in 30% of treatments. The advantages over hemodialysis are limited, though some poisons like paraquat and organophosphorus compounds may be effectively removed in early stages.

## PLASMA EXCHANGE

A process of limited use except for very high molecular weight toxins like monoclonal antibodies and to a lesser extent highly protein bound toxins like digoxin.

## TECHNICAL ASPECTS OF EXTRACORPOREAL TREATMENT OF POISONING

Cannulation of the femoral or internal jugular vein with a 12F or 14F cannula is required. Blood flow and dialysate flow in hemodialysis are variable, generally higher the blood flow higher the clearances. In hemoperfusion the blood flow is generally limited to 150–200 mL/min to allow adequate binding of toxin, but the anticoagulation requirements are higher with the activated partial thromboplastin time kept at twice the control value. In combination therapy the blood should first pass through the dialyzer and thereafter the hemoperfusion cartridge so that there is minimal saturation of the cartridge that increases its life span. A plasma filter may sometimes be used to separate plasma which is then run over a hemoperfusion cartridge and reinfused into the venous bubble chamber to limit the exposure of blood cells to the adsorption cartridge. These more complex arrangements are only required in a few specific situations.

Table 2 shows the available hemoperfusion devices with their characteristics.

### Initiating Extracorporeal Therapy

The decision to start extracorporeal therapy is usually made based on a combination of clinical signs, rate of deterioration, and the algorithm presented earlier. Plasma levels are available for a limited number of toxins and may be useful in aiding decision making, but frequently the time to obtain a report limits their use.

Table 3 summarizes the available evidence for some commonly occurring overdoses.

**Table 2:** Available hemoperfusion devices

| *Manufacturer* | *Device* | *Sorbent* | *Amount of sorbent* | *Polymer coating* |
|---|---|---|---|---|
| Asahi | Hemosorba | Bead charcoal | 170 g | Poly-Hema |
| Gambro | Adsorba | Norit (charcoal) | 100 or 300 g | Cellulose acetate |
| Braun | Hemoresin | XAD-4 | 350 g | None |
| Smith and Nephew | Hemocol | Sutcliffe Speakman charcoal | 100 or 300 g | Acrylic hydrogel |
| Clark | Biocompatible system | Charcoal | 50, 100, and 250 mL | Heparinized polymer |
| Organon-Teknika | Hemopur 260 | Norit extruded (Charcoal) | 260 g | Cellulose acetate |

**Table 3:** Available evidence for commonly occurring overdoses.

| *Drug* | *Indication for RRT* | *Serum concentration (mg/L)* | *Clearance without HD* | *Clearance with HD* | *RRT of Choice* |
|---|---|---|---|---|---|
| Methanol | pH <7.3<br>Methanol level >50 mg/dL<br>Visual changes, AKI<br>Severe electrolyte derangements<br>Hemodynamic instability and progression despite appropriate care | 500 | 11.3 mL/min | 125–215 mL/min | HD/SLED |
| Ethylene glycol | pH <7.3<br>Ethylene glycol level >50 mg/dL<br>Glycolic acid level >8 mmol/L<br>Refractory hyperosmolarity, AKI, severe electrolyte derangements<br>Hemodynamic instability and progression despite appropriate care | | Up to 27 | 145–230 | |
| Diethylene glycol | Hemodynamic instability and progression despite appropriate care<br>Persistent high anion gap acidosis | | Unknown | Unknown | |
| Isopropyl alcohol | Hemodynamic instability and progression despite appropriate care | >4,000 mg/dL | Unknown | 137 (isopropyl alcohol)<br>165 (acetone) | |
| Ethanol | | 100 | | | SLED |
| Aspirin | Serum level >90 mg/L<br>Severe acidosis<br>Neurologic symptoms, seizures, hyperthermia,<br>Acute respiratory distress syndrome (ARDS) | 800 | 0.6–25 mL/min | 3–100 mL/min | HD |
| Lithium | Serum level >2.5 mmol/L<br>Rising level<br>Renal insufficiency | 3.5 | 20–40 mL/min | 70–170 mL/min | HD |
| Valproate | Coma<br>Severe hepatic dysfunction | | 5–10 mL/min | 50–90 mL/min | HD |
| Metformin | Lactic acidosis | | 7 mL/min | Up to 170 mL/min | HD/SLED |
| Dabigatran | Bleeding especially intracranial | | Dependant on renal function | Decreases concentration by at least 40% | HD |
| Carbamazepine | Altered mental status<br>Seizures<br>Hemodynamic instability<br>Arrhythmias | | Supportive | Reduces level by about 50% | HD |

*Contd...*

*Contd...*

| *Drug* | *Indication for RRT* | *Serum concentration (mg/L)* | *Clearance without HD* | *Clearance with HD* | *RRT of Choice* |
|---|---|---|---|---|---|
| Phenobarbitone | Altered mental status | 100 | Supportive | Reduces level by about 60% in 4 hours | HD/ hemoperfusion |
| Phenytoin | Horizontal nystagmus<br>Ataxia<br>Altered mental status<br>Arrhythmias<br>Hypersensitivity reactions | | Supportive | Severe poisoning not responding to supportive care | HD |
| Diltiazem<br>Atenolol | Bradycardia<br>Hemodynamic instability | | Supportive | Unstable patient with renal failure not responding to supportive care | |
| Meprobamate | | 100 | | | Hemoperfusion |
| Paraquat | Very early onset multiorgan failure, lung fibrosis in late stages | 0.1 | | | Hemoperfusion superior to HD |
| Theophylline | Arrhythmias<br>Altered mental status<br>Seizures | 40 | Supportive | Unstable patient with renal failure not responding to supportive care | Hemoperfusion/ HD |
| Methaqualone | | 40 | | | Hemoperfusion |
| Cefepime | Neurotoxicity<br>Altered mental status | | Supportive | Unstable patient with renal failure not responding to supportive care | HD/CRRT |
| Acetaminophen | Liver failure | | Supportive<br>N-acetylcysteine<br>Liver transplant | Unstable patients with metabolic acidosis | HD/CRRT/SLED/ plasma exchange |

(AKI: acute kidney injury; ARDS: acute respiratory distress syndrome; CRRT: continuous renal replacement therapy; HD: hemodialysis; RRT: renal replacement therapy; SLED: sustained low-efficiency dialysis)

## SUMMARY

The role of extracorporeal therapies in poisoning may be limited but can be lifesaving or prevent crippling permanent organ damage (paraquat) in selected cases. The therapies should be used judiciously in cases and avoided where adequate supportive therapy or antidotes are possible. Access to drug levels or a toxin screen is useful especially if rapidly available in the case of consumption or exposure to an unknown toxin. Unavailability of levels should not lead to delay in initiating extracorporeal therapy in cases where the clinical situation warrants it especially where multiorgan involvement is present or imminent.

CHAPTER 18

# Nutrition for Acute Kidney Injury Patients on Renal Replacement Therapy

*Venkatesh Dhat*

## INTRODUCTION

Acute kidney injury (AKI) is associated with sudden decrease in the glomerular filtration rate with accumulation of the waste products, drugs, toxins, and altered functional capacity of the kidneys. Impairment in the kidney functions is variable and is based upon extent, magnitude, and duration of the AKI. It is common in the critically ill patients admitted to intensive care unit (ICU) and the incidence ranges from 20% to 60%.

It leads to various metabolic changes in macronutrients, and thus is responsible for hypercatabolic, pro-oxidative and proinflammatory state. And up to 50% of these AKI patients may need renal replacement therapy (RRT).

Acute renal failure in patients undergoing RRT presents an excess risk of in-hospital death.[8] The nutritional state of a patient at the initiation of dialysis is a clinically significant risk factor for mortality and morbidity on dialysis.[11]

## METABOLIC ALTERATIONS IN ACUTE KIDNEY INJURY

### Carbohydrate Metabolism

The most common derangement in carbohydrate metabolism is increased insulin resistance and hyperglycemia due to the action of catabolic hormones like glucagon, epinephrine, and cortisol. Patients with AKI are prone to exacerbated insulin resistance due to decreased renal gluconeogenesis and decreased hormonal clearances of insulin and glucagon.

### Lipid Metabolism

Increased plasma triglycerides, very low density lipoproteins, and low density lipoproteins are due to impaired lipolysis whereas the total circulating cholesterol and high density lipoprotein are decreased in AKI. Though the clearance of lipids is decreased in AKI, fatty acid oxidation is preserved so lipids remain an important energy source in these patients.

## Protein Metabolism

Acute kidney injury and critical illness both, if present, result in a prolonged intense state of protein catabolism. Metabolic acidosis in AKI, along with increased insulin resistance in critical illness, further promotes increased protein catabolism. Transport of amino acids into skeletal muscle is altered, and synthesis of proteins, other than visceral and acute phase proteins, is inhibited.

## Electrolytes

Acute kidney injury is also associated with major fluid, electrolyte, and acid-base derangements such as hypo or hypernatremia, hyperkalemia, hyperphosphatemia, and metabolic acidosis.

The pathogenesis of protein-energy wasting (PEW) in AKI is complex, and involves many different factors and mechanisms. PEW seems to be a frequent problem in AKI.

Many factors are likely to contribute to PEW in these patients, which include inadequate nutritional support, pre-existing poor nutritional status, superimposed catabolic illnesses (sepsis, trauma, surgery, chemotherapy, etc.), acidosis, blood losses, and nutrient losses during extracorporeal circulation, etc. Moreover, a key role is thought to be played by specific derangements in metabolic and hormonal pathways, leading to lean body mass catabolism.

Protein-energy wasting in AKI also increases risk for in-hospital complications and overall use of healthcare resources.

# ASSESSMENT OF THE NUTRITIONAL STATUS

Regular assessment of nutritional status in AKI patients and those requiring RRT is important and early detection of malnutrition can be helpful in improving this condition. Different methods are used in the evaluation of nutritional status in AKI patients. Biochemical and anthropometric measurements; nitrogen and energy balance techniques; record of food intake; subjective global assessment (SGA); bioimpedance analysis (BIA); dual-energy X-ray absorptiometry (DEXA); creatinine kinetics; neutron activation analysis and nuclear magnetic resonance spectrometry; serum markers: albumin, pre-albumin, insulin-like growth factor-1 (IGF-1), and transferrin; main proteins of the acute phase [C-reactive protein (CRP), serum amyloid A]; secondary proteins of the acute phase (fibrinogen, ferritin, complement); and cytokines [interleukin-6 (IL-6), tumor necrosis factor] are used to assess the nutritional status of patients with chronic renal failure.[5]

## Nutritional History

Nutritional history and dietary record provide information about nutrition of patients and enable us to determine those patients who are at risk of development of malnutrition

## Anthropometry

Anthropometry, a bedside test, is simple and inexpensive test used for nutritional assessment. This test includes estimation of percentage of weight loss, percentage of standard body weight, body mass index (BMI), and skin fold thickness at four sites.

Although measurements like arm circumference and skin fold thickness are used as representative of adipose and muscular tissue body compartments in several types of patients, their use in critically ill patients is very limited, since it seems to reflect more total body water rearrangement than modifications in body composition.[5]

## Body Mass Index

Body mass index is calculated by dividing weight in kg by square of the height in meters. BMI of less than 20 is associated with high mortality in AKI patients. BMI is not a perfect measure of body composition, since it is influenced by the presence of edema.

## Subjective Global Assessment

There are seven components to assess nutritional status; two components are related to physical examination (indicator of fat and muscle loss and nutritional status-associated with changes in fluid balance) and five components of medical history (weight change, diet, gastrointestinal symptoms, functional capacity, disease and nutrition relationship needs). While SGA scoring, points are given in each section of 1–7 and are categorized as 1–2 points (bad), 3–5 points (moderate), and 6–7 points (mild). Most of 3, 4 or 5 points show moderate malnutrition. Most of the findings of sections 1 or 2 points received are recognized as marked malnutrition and severe malnutrition.[5]

## Biochemical Markers for Nutritional Assessment (Table 1)

### *Albumin*

Lower levels of albumin have been associated with mortality.

Albumin is a negative acute phase protein, except nutritional status, and its synthesis is suppressed during inflammation. For this reason, there are limitations in the use of serum albumin level in order to assess the nutritional status of patients due to be affected by malnutrition and inflammatory reactions.

**Table 1:** Nutritional markers and their limitations in acute kidney injuries patients[6]

| | |
|---|---|
| Albumin, prealbumin, and cholesterol | May be reduced regardless of PEW (negative inflammation marker) |
| Body weight changes | Total body water is increased in AKI<br>Hypervolemia can mask changes in muscle mass |
| Anthropometry (triceps skin fold, arm circumference, etc.) | Influence by edema |
| Protien catabolic rate or protein equivalent of nitrogen emergence | Measurements require calculations based on urea kinetics during RRT + collection of dialysate |
| Nutrition score (SGA and its modifications ) | Most data are from patients with chronic renal patients. |
| Inflammatory markers (CRP, serum inerleukins, etc.) | Patient PEW prognostic/risk markers, non-<br>Useful FPR nutritional diagnosis and monitoring |

(AKI: acute kidney injury; PEW: protein energy wasting; CRP: c-reactive protein; SGA: subjective global assessment; RRT: renal replacement therapy)

Prealbumin is another marker. Because of the shorter half-life of prealbumin, many authors consider prealbumin to be a better marker of nutrition than serum albumin.

To assess the nutrition status of patients with AKI, the clinician must recognize the complications associated with the anthropometric markers, implementing good clinical judgment and an appreciation for the patient's history, presentation, and clinical course.

A major problem in AKI is the lack of adequate tools for nutritional status evaluation at the individual level, and for monitoring of the effects of nutritional support.

## EFFECT OF RENAL REPLACEMENT THERAPY ON NUTRITION

Dialysis increases nutrient losses and thus increases risk of PEW (Table 2).

In all cases, the losses depend on the frequency and duration of RRT, the membranes used, and the dialysate fluid's composition. The greatest losses occur with continuous renal replacement therapy (CRRT) and can be attributed to high ultrafiltrate volumes, use of filters with high permeability, and the continuous nature of the method.

In ICU patients with AKI, plasma levels of water-soluble vitamins, such as vitamin C, thiamine, and folic acid, may be lower than normal due mainly to the losses occurring through the RRT.

### Effects of Continuous Renal Replacement Therapy

With CRRT, 10–15% of infused amino acids are lost every day (up to 15–20% in the case of glutamine, 0.5–6.8 g/day when supplementation is 0.32 g/kg/day).

Apart from decrease in uremic intoxication, CRRT causes loss of heat/energy, loss of substrates like amino acids and vitamins, intake of some substrates like lactate, citrate, and glucose, elimination of short-chained peptides like cytokines, activation of mediator cascades, and stimulation of protein catabolism.

Continuous renal replacement therapy also causes various electrolyte disorders (sodium, potassium, magnesium, and phosphate) and induction of metabolic alkalosis.

## NUTRITIONAL REQUIREMENT

Enteral nutrition (EN) is the preferred method of nutrition delivery in AKI patients with a functioning intestine.

**Table 2:** Nutrient losses during renal replacement therapy.[9]

| *Nutrient* | *Hemodialysis* | *CRRT* | *Peritoneal dialysis* |
|---|---|---|---|
| Amino acids | 6–12 g/session | 10–15 g/day | 2–4 g/day |
| Proteins | 0.5–15 g/session | 5–10 g/day | 5–15 g/day |
| Glucose | 25 g/session with glucose—free dialysate; no loss with glucose-based dialysate | Unknown | Uptake of 100–150 g/day |

Note: RRT can be associated with the loss of up to 10–20 g amino acids in each session, depending on RRT modality and filter type.

Parenteral nutrition (PN) should be reserved for those patients who are unable to tolerate EN or if EN does not meet their energy and protein requirements.

## Goals of Nutrition

The goals of nutrition support in patients with AKI are consistent with the goals for critically ill patients and include delivery of energy, protein, and micronutrients to:

- Prevent PEW
- Preservation of lean body mass
- Maintenance of nutrition status
- Avoidance of further metabolic derangements
- Enhancement of wound healing
- Support of immune function
- Attenuation of the patients' inflammatory status.

## Energy Requirement

Energy delivery in patients with AKI is recommended from 25 kcal/kg/day to 35 kcal/kg/day.

Nutrition support should be based on estimated metabolic stress and protein energy requirements.

Higher caloric delivery has been studied but does not appear to improve patient outcomes.

## Protein Requirement

Daily protein intake should be in the range of 1.2–1.7 g/kg actual body weight in AKI patients.

Provision of adequate nonprotein calories should be maintained to achieve total energy intake in patients with AKI.

Recommendations for protein delivery in patients with AKI receiving RRT range from 1.5 g/kg/day to 2.5 g/kg/day and depend on the patient's severity of AKI, the underlying disease states and complications, and the type of RRT employed.

A significant amino acid loss (10–15 g/day) is associated with CRRT. Thus, patients on this therapy may require at least an additional 0.2 g/kg/day totaling up to 2.5 g/kg/day. No major advantages have been demonstrated with very high protein intakes (>2.5 g/kg/day), as excessively high nitrogen intakes may simply increase the rate of urea production.[1,2]

## Carbohydrates

Estimated glucose requirement per day is 5–7 g/kg/day.

## Lipid Requirement

The recommendations for lipids range from 0.7 g/kg/day to 1.5 g/kg/day. Some recommend the use of about 30% or one-third of total non-protein calories, both using lipid emulsions composed of medium- and long-chain triglycerides. Since fatty acid oxidation is decreased in AKI, serum triglycerides should be closely monitored, and the administration of the diet should be discontinued whenever their levels exceed 400 mg/dL.

## Micronutrients

### *Vitamin A*

The intake of dietary vitamin A for AKI patients on RRT should not exceed 800–1,000 mg/day.

### *Vitamin B Complex*

Thiamine is the micronutrient at the highest risk of depletion during RRT. An additional 100 mg of thiamine should be intravenously delivered daily while patients are receiving CRRT.

Vitamin B6 and folic acid intake in hemodialysis (HD) patients are higher than normal healthy subjects.

### *Vitamin C*

The required amount of vitamin C in patients with AKI is 50–100 mg/day; higher intakes (up to 150–200 mg) may be needed when CRRT is used.[7]

### *Vitamin E*

Increased oxidative stress and cardiovascular risks are associated with RRT patients. The antioxidant properties of vitamin E may be useful in preventing or reducing these risks. HD patients are recommended a daily intake of 400 IU of vitamin E.

### *Phosphorus*

Patients receiving CRRT typically have hypophosphatemia and require supplemental phosphorus. It can be replaced as per the need. Severe hypophosphatemia has been associated with respiratory muscle weakness, phosphate depletion, ventilator failure, myocardial dysfunction, and encephalopathy in critically ill patients; moreover, a higher incidence of prolonged respiratory failure requiring tracheostomy has been documented in patients with AKI on continuous RRT.

### *Trace Elements*

Renal replacement therapy fluids (dialysis fluid or replacement fluid) may have variable content of trace elements, at concentrations often difficult to detect; the effects of RRT on the removal of mainly protein-bound trace elements are far from being clearly defined. Some studies indicate that selenium, chromium, copper, and zinc can be removed from plasma by convective/diffusive RRTs.[7]

Thus, patients with AKI on RRT are at risk of trace element depletion.

Zinc, iron, magnesium (Mg)—15 mg/day, 10–18 mg/day, 200–300 mg/day are needed, respectively, in patients who are on RRT.

Selenium deficiencies have been found in patients receiving CRRT with deficits estimated from 35 μg/day to 91 μg/day. Losses of selenium via CRRT result in deficiency if not corrected. An additional 100 μg/day of selenium in addition to the standard multiple trace element preparation is recommended.

*Copper:* 400 μg of copper is lost during CRRT, and hence an intake of 300–500 μg/day is recommended.

## TOTAL PARENTERAL NUTRITION IN ACUTE KIDNEY INJURY ON RENAL REPLACEMENT THERAPY

Indications of PN are similar to the indications for PN in nonrenal patients:

- Malnourished patients requiring nutritional support should be considered for PN when oral nutritional supplements (ONS) and EN are impossible or fail to reach nutritional goals.
- When nutritional requirements cannot be met by dietary intake (with or without ONS), in combination with EN or by the enteral route alone.

Standard formulae for PN (amino acids solutions and commercial three-in-one nutrient admixtures) containing both essential and nonessential amino acids are preferred in AKI on RRT.

In some patients, three in one nutrient admixtures without electrolytes (i.e. without sodium, potassium, etc.) are now commercially available, and can be used with caution and careful monitoring or customized according to patient needs. Whether immune enhancing diets should be given to AKI patients remains unsettled (Table 3).[10]

**Table 3:** Recommended dietary nutrient intake for AKI patients who require RRT[5]

| | |
|---|---|
| Dietary protein intake | 1.2 -1.5 g/kg/day |
| Daily energy intake (DEI ) | 25–35 kcal/d |
| Total fat | 25–35 % of total energy intake |
| Carbohydrates | Rest of the calories |
| Total fiber | >20–25 g/day |
| Sodium | 750–200 mg/day |
| Potassium | 2000–2750 mg/day |
| Phosphorus | 800–1000 mg/day |
| Calcium | <1000 mg/day |
| Magnesium | 200–300 mg/day |
| Selenium | 55 ug/day |
| Water | Usually 750–1500 mL/d |
| Vitamin $B_1$ | 1.1–1.2 mg/d |
| Vitamin $B_2$ | 1.1–1.3 mg/day |
| Biotin | 30 μg/day |
| Niacin | 14–16 mg/day |
| Vitamin $B_6$ | 10 mg/day |
| Vitamin $B_{12}$ | 24 μg/day |
| Vitamin C | 75–90 mg/day |
| Folic Acid | 1–5 mg/day. |
| Vitamin A | 800-1000 μg/day |
| Vitamin D | 1000–1500 IU |
| Vitamin E | 400–800/IU |

## SUMMARY

- Acute kidney injury in the critically ill patient rarely occurs as an isolated organ failure, occurring during severe and often prolonged catabolic phases of the critical illness.
- Patients who develop AKI often have pre-existing or hospital-acquired protein-energy malnutrition, which is a major negative prognostic factor in this patient.
- The primary goals of nutritional support in AKI are the same as those for other critically ill patients with normal renal function, i.e. to ensure the delivery of adequate nutrition, to prevent PEW with its attendant metabolic complications, to promote wound healing and tissue repair, to support immune system function, to accelerate recovery, and to reduce mortality.
- For nutritional support, the enteral route is preferred, although it often needs to be supplemented by the parenteral route in order to meet nutritional requirements.
- Due to the loss of the kidney's homeostatic function and need of renal replacement therapy, patients with acute kidney injury are in a high risk of complications related to the nutritional status such as hyperglycemia, hypertriglyceridemia, fluid retention, and electrolyte and acid-base disorders.
- Nutritional requirements should be frequently reassessed, individualized, and carefully integrated with RRT.
- Patients with AKI on RRT should receive a basic intake of at least 1.5 g/kg/day of protein with an additional 0.2 g/kg/day to compensate for protein lost during RRT. Energy intake should consist of no more than 30 calories.[1,2]
- The type of CRRT procedure, the membrane used, the type of anticoagulation, and the characteristics of the replacement fluid (i.e. composition and placement of replacement fluid) and/or dialysate can all influence these recommendations.

## REFERENCES


1. Mehta Y, Sunavala JD, Zirpe K, et al. Practice Guidelines for Nutrition in Critically Ill Patients: A Relook for Indian Scenario. Indian J Crit Care Med. 2018;22(4):263-73.
2. McClave SA, Taylor BE, Martindale RG, et al. Guidelines for the Provision and Assessment of Nutrition Support Therapy in the Adult Critically Ill Patient: Society of Critical Care Medicine (SCCM) and American Society for Parenteral and Enteral Nutrition (A.S.P.E.N.). JPEN J Parenter Enteral Nutr. 2016;40(2):159-211.
3. Gervasio JM, Garmon WP, Holowatyj M. Nutrition support in acute kidney Injury. Scholarship and Professional Work – COPHS. Paper 3. 2011.
4. Fiaccadori E, Regolisti G, Maggiore U. Specialized Nutritional support interventions in critically ill patients on renal replacement therapy. Curr Opin Clin Nutr Metab Care. 2013;16(2):217-24.
5. Güneş FE. Medical nutrition therapy for hemodialysis patients. In: Suzuki H (Ed). Hemodialysis. UK: IntechOpen; 2013.
6. Berbel MN, Pinto MPR, Ponce D, et al. Nutritional aspects in acute kidney injury. Rev Assoc Med Bras. 2011;57(5):587-92.
7. Fiaccadori E, Regolisti G, Cabassi A. Specific nutritional problems in acute kidney injury, treated with non-dialysis and dialytic modalities. NDT Plus. 2010;3:1-7.

8. Metnitz PG, Krenn CG, Steltzer H, et al. Effect of acute renal failure requiring renal replacement therapy on outcome in critically ill patients. Crit Care Med. 2002;30(9):2051-8.
9. Lindholm B, Wang T, Heimbürger O, et al. Influence of different treatments and schedules on the factors conditioning the nutritional status in dialysis patients. Nephrol Dial Transplant. 1998;13: 66-73.
10. Cano NJ, Aparicio M, Brunori G, et al. ESPEN Guidelines on Parenteral Nutrition: adult renal failure. Clin Nutr. 2009;28(4):401-14.
11. K/DOQI Clinical Practice Guidelines. Am J Kidney Dis. 2000;35(6).

CHAPTER 19

# Renal Replacement Therapy in ICU: Infection Control and Prevention

*Sushma Gurav, Kapil Zirpe*

## INTRODUCTION

End-stage renal disease (ESRD) patients and dialysis unit staff are susceptible for infectious diseases due to frequent exposure to pathogens. Patients requiring regular dialysis [hemodialysis (HD)] are susceptible to various types of infections: bloodstream infections and localized infections of vascular access; blood-borne infections with hepatitis B virus (HBV), hepatitis C virus, and/or human immunodeficiency virus (HIV); and airborne infections. Infection is the first cause of hospitalization and the second most common cause of mortality among the patients requiring dialysis. Thus the need to initiate infection prevention and control program should at earliest.[1]

Centers for Disease Control and Prevention (CDC) estimates 37,000 central line-associated bloodstream infections may have occurred in US hemodialysis patients in 2008 (MMWR, 2011).

## EPIDEMIOLOGY OF INFECTIONS AMONG HEMODIALYSIS PATIENTS

Infections are the second leading cause of death. Various sites of infection in these patients are:[2]

- 57% vascular access
- 23% wound
- 15% lung
- 5% urinary tract.

## TYPES OF INFECTIONS IN HEMODIALYSIS UNIT

- *Infections due to the process of hemodialysis:*
  - Catheter-related bacteremia, infective endocarditis, and metastatic septic emboli
  - Arteriovenous fistula/arteriovenous graft (AVF/AVG) infections
  - Dialysate water-related infections.
- *Infectious transmission between patients:*
  - Hepatitis B and C and HIV

- Methicillin-resistant *Staphylococcus aureus* carrier state
- *Respiratory infections:* Tuberculosis, influenza, and pneumococcal.

## WHY ESRD PATIENTS ARE AT INCREASED RISK OF INFECTION?

Following are the reasons for increased risk of infection:[1]

- Immune-compromised status of dialysis patients
- Frequent and prolonged blood exposure during hemodialysis through vascular access (mainly catheters) and extracorporeal circuit (with many ports and connections)
- Contact with other patients during treatment
- Frequent contact with healthcare workers, who frequently move between patients and between machines
- Frequent hospitalization and requirement of surgeries
- Nonadherence or breaks in implementation of infection control policies
- Comorbidities, high rates of hospitalisation, and high rates of antibiotic exposure make these patients have high prevalence rate of colonization with multiresistant organisms.[3]

## SOURCES OF INFECTIONS IN DIALYSIS UNIT

Sources of infections in dialysis unit are: contaminated water, equipment, environmental surfaces, infected patients, and contaminated healthcare worker hands. Among these, most common mode of transmission for healthcare-associated infections is the contaminated hands of healthcare provider.[1]

Following are the three elements required for an infection to occur:

1. A *source* of germs (like bacteria or viruses or fungal)
2. A susceptible *host/media*, meaning a person who is at risk of getting an infection from the germs or a media for growth of organism.
3. A *way/mode* for the germs to move from the source to the host:
   - Three ways in which germs move from the source to the host are: *contact, droplet, and airborne transmission.*

   During dialysis, infections are commonly spread by *contact transmission*. As stated earlier *Healthcare worker hands!*[4-7] *are the most common mode/way of spreading infection*

Most important step in infection prevention for each dialysis unit or hospitals is to develop and implement an infection control program. The infection prevention and management program should also include:

- Infection surveillance and monitoring processes, strategy development to reduce or minimize the risk of infection, and evaluation and feedback processes, i.e. audits should be conducted assessing the pitfalls and thereafter redesigning and implementing the revised program. Dialysis units should also form a rapid response team for emergencies such as epidemics and national disasters related to infectious diseases.[1,5-7]

The areas of infection control covered in dialysis unit include: standard precautions, isolation strategies, vascular access care, water treatment, cleaning/disinfecting/sterilizing, vaccination, and infection prevention and control program.[6,7]

## STANDARD PRECAUTIONS

Suggested "Standard Precautions" that need to be followed by all healthcare workers are:[5-7]

- Hand hygiene techniques
- Compulsory use of personal protective equipment (PPE)
- Follow safe injection practices
- Vaccination of dialysis staff and patients
- Preventing the spread of hepatitis B
- Preventing the spread of bacterial infections.

Hand hygiene is the simplest and most important technique in prevention of infection. It should be practised:

- *Before*: Before touching a patient, before performing a clean or aseptic procedure, before intervention (e.g. dialysis preparation), before drug administration, before management of an area with broken skin integrity (e.g. catheter dressing), and before an invasive procedure.
- *After*: After touching (e.g. measurement of vital signs) a patient, after exposure to body fluid (e.g. hemostasis after dialysis therapy), after touching a patient's surroundings (e.g. bed, bedsheets of patient).

Relatives and visitors must perform hand hygiene in an appropriate manner when entering the dialysis room.

Staff training, hand hygiene, vascular access care audits, and staff feedback result in a significant reduction in access-related bloodstream infections. To improve adherence use of checklists and monthly audits of hand hygiene practices and a feedback system to the caregivers are strongly recommended.[4]

## INFECTION CONTROL FOR VASCULAR ACCESS

A vascular access helps to move blood from the patient to the hemodialysis machine. There are three kinds of access: fistulas, grafts, and central line catheters. Central line catheters are associated with increased infections rates compared to grafts or fistulas. A fistula generally lasts longer and has fewer problems such as infections and clotting.

### Dialysis Catheter Insertion

Temporary dialysis catheters should be kept for a minimum period and removed at the earliest. If it is not possible to establish arteriovenous fistulae for 1–2 weeks, a tunneled catheter with a cuff should be inserted. Aseptic techniques should be followed during insertion of vascular cannulae. The procedure should be performed by well-trained medical staff. Recommended maximum barrier precautions are a surgical mask, a sterilized gown, sterilized gloves, a cap, and a whole-body drape should be used for catheter insertion.

The site of catheter insertion should be disinfected with a 0.5–2% chlorhexidine/alcohol solution. In order to prevent catheter-related complications, internal jugular vein is the preferred site for catheter insertion. The femoral and subclavian veins site should be avoided if possible.

To reduce the number of attempts and complications ultrasound can be used to identify a vein during the insertion of a hemodialysis catheter.[6,7]

### Catheter Exit-site Care

Before each hemodialysis session catheter exit-site and catheter hub should be examined for any infection.

At the time of changing of dressing, the skin at catheter exit should be cleaned with 2% chlorhexidine/70% alcohol or a 10% povidone-iodine solution. Few essential steps in infection prevention are routine performance of catheter hub disinfection ("scrub the hub") and applying antimicrobial ointment or chlorhexidine impregnated dressing to the catheter exit-site. Antimicrobial barrier caps are also available and these caps can help to reduce catheter-related bloodstream infections and are widely used.[4,6,7]

The employee should wear a mask and sterile gloves while manipulating the catheter. The dressing should be changed before each hemodialysis session if it is a gauze-type dressing. If it is a transparent dressing, it should be changed every 7 days or else whenever the dressing is wet or soiled.

## INFECTION PREVENTION DURING THE DIALYSIS

Hand hygiene and aseptic techniques are the most effective steps to be followed throughout all dialysis procedures.[6,7]

Any item taken to a patient's dialysis station could have become contaminated.

- Items taken to the dialysis station should either be:
  - Disposed, or
  - Cleaned and disinfected before being taken to a common clean area or used on another patient.

Unused medications or medicine vials (e.g. medication vials, syringes, alcohol swabs) taken to the patient's station should not be returned to a common clean area.

Centers for Disease Control and Prevention recommends that use single-dose vials whenever possible and dispose of them immediately after use. Prepare the medication in a clean area/room away from the patient station. It should be brought to the patient station only at the time of use.

For the preparation of multidose injections, e.g. heparin, each dose should be weighed in a separate syringe for each patient in the preparation room, and multidose injection vials should not be taken to the patient treatment area. The multidose vial should be stored in a refrigerator at 2°C to 8°C until subsequent use. The rubber diaphragm should be disinfected before every use.

### Control of the Source of Blood-borne Infections[6,7]

Main aim of infection control program is to prevent blood-borne infection.

All patients who need hemodialysis should be routinely screened for hepatitis B and hepatitis C infections. Patients who are at risk for developing hepatitis B infection should be vaccinated against HBV.

### Care of HBsAg Positive Patients

Separate machines, equipment, instruments, and supplies should be used to dialyze hepatitis B antigen (HBsAg) positive patient. An HBsAg-positive patient should be taken care by a dedicated nurse/healthcare provider. This nurse should not take care of patients who are at risk for infection (anti-HBs negative) at the same time. The dialysis membranes used for HBsAg-positive patients should not be reused because as the employees may get infected while cleaning of the filter.

### Care of HIV and HCV Positive Patients

Patients with negative anti-HCV results should undergo anti-HCV testing every 6 months. Regular HIV testing is not recommended for infection control purposes.

If standard precautions are followed, hepatitis C and HIV positive patients need not to be isolated from other patients or dialyzed with separate dedicated machines.

### Care of Patients with Bacterial Infections

Hemodialysis patients who might be at increased risk for spreading germs to other patients include those with:

- An infected skin wound with drainage that is not contained by dressings.
- Fecal incontinence or uncontrolled diarrhea.
- With respiratory illness and a fever are at risk of spreading bacterial and viral respiratory infections.

For these patients use the following precautions:

- Wear a gown and gloves (PPE) when you are caring for the patient and discard the gown and gloves after caring for the patient is done.
- Do not wear the same gown when caring for other patients.
- Dialyze the patient at a station with as few adjacent stations as possible (e.g. at the end or corner of the room).

## VACCINATION

Staff and healthcare provider should get vaccinated:

- Flu vaccine each year
- Complete the hepatitis B vaccine schedule.

## WATER TREATMENT[6,7]

The depending upon degree of purification of water used for dialysis, water used for dialysis is labelled as standard pure water or ultrapure water. The use of ultrapure water is considered important during hemodialysis, specifically in the case of high-flux dialysis or hemodiafiltration.

The steps in water purification are preprocessing (microfilter, softener, and carbon filter), reverse osmosis (RO), deionizing, and postprocessing procedures. Water produced for dialysis is tested regularly for bacteriological and chemical contaminants. Two samples of water are to be sent for assay. One sample of water is to be taken from the RO port before dialysis, and second sample is taken from the sampling port of the hemodialysis machine during or after dialysis. If the assay report of tested water exceeds acceptable levels, corrective measures should be taken promptly to reduce the levels of bacteria/chemicals. To evaluate the adequacy of disinfection process of the dialysis machine, the bacteriological assays of water should be performed weekly in the beginning and then should be done monthly once the process has been established. Endotoxin assays should be performed every 3 months, or more frequently if the water treatment system is being tested for adequacy. Chemical assay of water used for dialysis is to done annually.

## WASTE MANAGEMENT[6,7]

The materials, such as the dialysis membranes, lines, or needles, used during hemodialysis process forms biomedical wastes. This biomedical waste should be placed in a special container, and handled by a waste disposal contractor. Hemodialysis fluid is not considered biomedical waste as it does not come into direct contact with blood.

## STERILIZING, DISINFECTING, AND CLEANING[4,6,7]

The equipment and items used in the dialysis process should be cleaned, disinfected, and sterilized as per their characteristics. Sterile equipment required in dialysis unit is stored at proper place and need to be used before expiry date. Dialysis unit should have dedicated separate area for cleaning and disinfecting nondisposable items used during dialysis. If these items need to be sterilized, then they are to be sent to sterile processing department. The healthcare provider needs to wear PPE while disinfecting the nondisposable items. Disposable items should be placed in medical waste containers after using them:

- Before removing or transporting used dialyzers and blood tubing, cap dialyzer ports and clamp tubing.
- Place all used dialyzers and tubing in leak-proof containers for transport from station to reprocessing or disposal area.

If dialyzers are reused, follow published methods (*the Association for the Advancement of Medical Instrumentation—AAMI).*

The water treatment and distribution system should be regularly disinfected according to the manufacturer's manual.

### Laundry Care[6,7]

Clean linens and cloths should be stored in separate place. Dialysis unit should have area for collection of laundry. Collected laundry is classified as contaminated laundry or other laundry. "Contaminated laundry" is linen used by an infected person or probably the linen was contaminated with body fluids (blood, pus, etc.) or infectious materials. Contaminated laundry should be collected in a separate laundry basket.

### Environmental Control[6,7]

Inadequately cleaned and disinfected dialysis stations, priming buckets, HD machines, effluent drain wall box, and other equipment are sources for transmission of pathogens in HD facilities.

Patient area, visitors or relatives waiting area, and employee area should be kept clean and safe. The hemodialysis machine should be rinsed after each dialysis session, and the interior of the dialysis machine should be disinfected at the end of the day. The surface of the hemodialyzer should be disinfected after each dialysis session with an ammonium compound or sodium hypochlorite at a 1:100 dilution. There should be a devoted "Waste treatment area" in the dialysis unit. The floor of the hemodialysis unit should be cleaned every day, or more frequently if it has been soiled or contaminated.

## STRATEGIES TO IMPROVE ADHERENCE[6]

Involving patients and their family members in infection control program will help to achieve 100% target in infection control program. Medical directors should actively collaborate with the nurse manager to perform staff audits of infection control measures, such as HD catheter care and sterile techniques for cannulating the vascular access. Physicians should engage their patients in infection control measures and encourage patients to speak up and ask questions without fear about infection control. Medical directors can minimize this risk by developing and implementing an antimicrobial stewardship program.

## EDUCATING PATIENTS AND THEIR CAREGIVERS[5-7]

### How to Recognize an Infection?

Advise patients to contact healthcare provider doctor if they notice any of the following possible signs of infection:

- Fever
- *The access site is:*
  - Swollen (bulging), red, warm, or has pus
- Severe pain at the access site.

When a new patient starts dialysis and on an annual basis, review:

- Personal hygiene and hand hygiene technique
- Patient responsibility for proper care of the access site and recognition of signs of infection
- Recommended vaccinations (including hepatitis B, influenza, and pneumococcal)
- Reasons for selecting a fistula or graft over a catheter to lower the risk of infection.

The factors responsible for difficulties in the implementation of recommended practices:[1,4]

- Understaffing with poor nurse-to-patient ratio
- Frequent turnover of nursing staff
- Lack or inadequate training and lower level of competency among HD staff
- Inadequate or lack of patient/family education
- Inadequate provision of necessary supplies/equipment
- Poor design of HD unit layout (congested and inadequate segregation/isolation)
- Life-threatening situation in dialysis unit may lead to divergence of standard precautions.

## REFERENCES

1. Karkar A. Infection control guidelines in hemodialysis facilities. Kidney Res Clin Pract. 2018;37(1):1-3.
2. Tokars JI, Miller ER, Stein G. United States Renal Data System: USRDS 2005 Annual Data Report: Atlas of End-Stage Renal Disease in the United States, Bethesda, National Institutes of Health, National Institute of Diabetes and Digestive and Kidney Diseases, 2005
3. Jardine M, Commons RJ, de Zoysa JR, et al. Kidney Health Australia. Caring for Australasians with Renal Impairment guideline recommendations for infection control for haemodialysis units. Nephrology (Carlton); 2018. [Epub ahead of print]
4. Vijayan A, Boyce JM. 100% Use of infection control procedures in hemodialysis facilities: call to action. Clin J Am Soc Nephrol. 2018;13(4):671-3.
5. CDC. Dialysis safety. [online] Available from http:/www.cdc.gov/dialysis [Last accessed June, 2019].
6. Karkar A, Bouhaha BM, Dammang ML. Infection control in hemodialysis units: a quick access to essential elements. Saudi J Kidney Dis Transpl. 2014;25(3):496-519.
7. Park HC, Lee YK, Yoo KD, et al. Korean clinical practice guidelines for preventing the transmission of infections in hemodialysis facilities. Kidney Res Clin Pract. 2018;37(1):8-19.

# Index

Page numbers followed by *b* refer to box, *f* refer to figure, and *t* refer to table

## A



## B